STRENGTH TRAINING FOR GOLFERS

ALSO BY JOHN LITTLE

Advanced Max Contraction Training
Beginning Bodybuilding
High Intensity Training the Mike Mentzer Way (with Mike Mentzer)
Max Contraction Training
One More Rep! (with Robert Wolff)
Power Factor Training (with Peter Sisco)
Static Contraction Training (with Peter Sisco)
The Wisdom of Mike Mentzer (with Joanne Sharkey)

STRENGTH TRAINING FOR GOLFERS

A Proven Regimen to Improve Your Strength, Flexibility, Endurance, and Distance Off the Tee

John Little

Foreword by Cary Howe

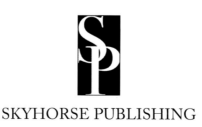

SKYHORSE PUBLISHING

Skyhorse Publishing books may be purchased in bulk at special discounts for sales promotion, corporate gifts, fund-raising, or educational purposes. Special editions can also be created to specifications. For details, contact the Special Sales Department, Skyhorse Publishing, 307 West 36th Street, 11th Floor, New York, NY 10018 or info@skyhorsepublishing.com.

Skyhorse® and Skyhorse Publishing® are registered trademarks of Skyhorse Publishing, Inc.®, a Delaware corporation.

Visit our website at www.skyhorsepublishing.com.

10 9 8 7 6 5 4 3 2 1

Library of Congress Cataloging-in-Publication Data is available on file.

ISBN: 978-1-61608-730-2

Printed in China

This book and the information contained herein is for education and entertainment purposes only and does not advocate or prescribe a specific exercise or nutritional plan for anyone, regardless of age, sex, or experience level.

Like all bodybuilding, exercise, fitness, health, and nutrition books, we strongly advise that you get the approval of a qualified medical/health authority before beginning any exercise program or making any dietary changes. The authors, publisher, people featured, or anyone associated with this book in any way shall not be held liable for anyone's actions either directly or indirectly.

DEDICATION

This book is dedicated to my wife, Terri, and to our children, Riley, Taylor, Brandon, and Benjamin, who encouraged me in the research, experimentation, and development of this protocol. It is also dedicated to my late father, William T. Little, who first introduced me to the game of golf (alas, when I was too young to appreciate it) and to Sally and Gord Sisco, who reintroduced me to the game many decades later. And finally, this book is dedicated to those individuals who value reason and science in their training and do not follow the "herd" mentality that so dominates popular culture.

FOREWORD

When I first walked through the doors of Nautilus North Strength and Fitness Centre in 2004, I was "green" by fitness industry standards to the whole concept of strength training. Although I had read many books on strength training and had played sports and trained with weights for years, I had no way of knowing that there was a "right" way and a "wrong" way of exercising—and that I (and most everyone else) had apparently been misled by the industry into thinking that there were only "different" ways. I worked with John Little from that year to the present and we agreed to test everything—every workout protocol, every recovery interval, every nutritional consideration that we had heard about. As a result, many concepts that were popular were found to be without foundation, and a new direction began to emerge.

We conducted studies on protocols to test training theories on large numbers of people to see what worked, to what degree it worked, and whether or not better results could be obtained. As someone who likes to golf, my interest in how to improve my game was always in the back of my mind. Many of the clients I train are also golfers and are hungry for knowledge on ways to improve their games as well. What taking part in all of these studies gave was an objective view of the data. Neither I nor my clients cared about the fitness industry, or what was the new hot trend. Instead, we wanted results—the quicker the better—and if that meant we didn't have to be in the gym three to four days a week, that was fine by us as we'd rather be out golfing anyway.

In the first year that I worked for John and Terri Little I personally supervised some 7,500 workouts and our facility oversaw some 25,000 workouts. Indeed, since we kept workout records on all of our clients there was already a considerable database of cause and effect relationships prior to setting out to conduct our more formal studies into the effects of exercise.

One of our first studies involved devising a means to determine an individual's optimal training frequency. For instance, when did the body produce a change in muscle mass and at what point would it begin to lose size after it had been produced? The results were astonishing. The first few days following the workout revealed to us that a trainee is not stronger, but weaker. Indeed, since recovery precedes growth, the data revealed that a trainee is not ready to work out again and would not make any meaningful progress for at least a week after a workout. We also discovered that, despite what the fitness industry has been saying for years, one did not lose what one had gained if one did not work out again within ninety-six hours. With help of the Bod Pod body composition testing machine, we were able to scientifically track what happens to the body in the two weeks after a high intensity workout—this was the first time that such a test had been performed.

Then we wanted to see how much fat could be lost in a ten-week period. Again, this had relevance to the game of golf as muscle is what contracts (not fat) and it is muscular contraction that moves the clubs. However, we had seen that the fitness industry belief was that you had to spend multiple hours over multiple days per week in order to lose body fat. Was this true? Or was there a better, simpler way? These were questions we wanted answers for when we conducted our second study. The answers to these questions will surprise you and are laid out in this book. The combined time of all ten workouts is less than what most personal trainers would have you go through in your first session. This study not only will change how people look at fat loss but it also spoke to how little training is actually required to accomplish it.

By reading this book and following the training guidelines you will become a stronger athlete, and a stronger athlete is a better athlete. Will it bring you up to the upper levels of the PGA? Probably not, but it will certainly allow you to better your own game and allow you to chase that little white ball much longer and to hit it a hell of a lot farther—without living your life in the gym.

—Cary Howe
Lead trainer, Nautilus North Strength & Fitness Centre
Bracebridge, Ontario

INTRODUCTION: TOWARDS A NEW PERSPECTIVE

To begin, it should be pointed out that this is not a golf book. It will not at any point speak of how to grip a club, how to position your feet, the arc of the swing, graphite clubs, or the "inner game" of golf. It is assumed that the reader already has some knowledge of these facets of the game, and presently is looking for a means of improving his overall strength and fitness levels so as to be able to improve upon his ability to play the game of golf more efficiently and with greater power.

However, this is not merely a compendium of workout routines. Instead, within these pages you will learn of a revolutionary new perspective on strength training. It is so revolutionary (at least compared to what is being typically served up as strength training for golfers) that you will need to open your mind to new facts and, surprising as this may sound, common sense. To help the reader cultivate the correct mindset for learning, I have reworked a short Zen parable.

A golfer once learned that a new training protocol had been developed that had produced fast and startling improvement in one's golf game. As the innovator of this protocol lived in semi-seclusion in a northern town, he decided he would make the trip to speak with him. The innovator received the golfer graciously and invited him out onto his deck on a beautiful summer day to answer his questions.

"Tell me about this system of yours," began the golfer. As the innovator began to explain, he was frequently interrupted by the golfer: "Oh, yes, in the gym where I work out, my personal trainer has me do something like that," and "it sounds interesting in theory but nobody I know trains that way." After several fruitless attempts to explain himself uninterrupted, the innovator finally suggested that they have a cup of coffee. The golfer agreed. The innovator went into his home and came out with a pot of coffee and two cups. He poured his own and then began to fill the golfer's cup. As the golfer continued to talk about the traditions and methods of the sports greatest champions, the innovator kept filling his cup until it began to overflow. "What are you doing?" asked the golfer incredulously. "Can't you see that the cup is full?" "Precisely," answered the innovator. "Like this cup, you are so full of your own preconceptions, opinions and traditions, that there is no more room in your mind for what I have to say. Unless you first empty your cup, how will you ever taste my cup of coffee?" The golfer got the point.

I would ask that you, like the golfer, first "empty your cup" of all preconceived notions, opinions, and traditions on the subject of how to train for the game of golf so that you will have room—intellectually—for what I am about to relate.

Anatomists tell us that more than four hundred muscles are responsible for allowing us to go about our daily activities. It's also common knowledge that if we don't make an effort to use them to 100 percent of their energy potential, they'll slowly wither away with the passage of time. Ironically, while all of us possess the same number of muscles, not all of us possess the same number of muscle fibers in each of our muscle groups. This explains why few of us can ever develop our muscles (not that many of us wish to) to the same size as champion bodybuilders. Let it be understood that the champions of any sport—whether of yesteryear, today, and, for that matter, tomorrow possessed one quality that the vast majority of us do not—uncommon genetics. The strongest and most muscular among them had long muscle bellies, greater muscle fiber density, greater than average bone thickness, and higher than normal metabolisms. However, while only a certain portion of the population can develop a heavy musculature, everyone can improve their strength and the size of their muscles to a considerable degree, along with dramatically improving their performance in the game of golf—if they train intelligently, scientifically, and realistically.

For years golfers seeking to become stronger have known that weight training is the key. However, how to best employ weights in developing maximum strength and realizing one's full muscular potential has been a rather foggy area at best. This book is an attempt to bring some much-needed science into the arena of strength training with the specific goal of improving one's golf game. For decades there has been the belief that if one merely aped a particular golfing champion's training method, then one could dramatically improve one's game—a belief that has been found to be completely erroneous.

This is not to suggest that there isn't a way to improve such aspects of the game as the power of your drive, better control of your irons, and improved precision in putting. There is. However, it has little or nothing to do with such things as stretching, mental concentration exercises

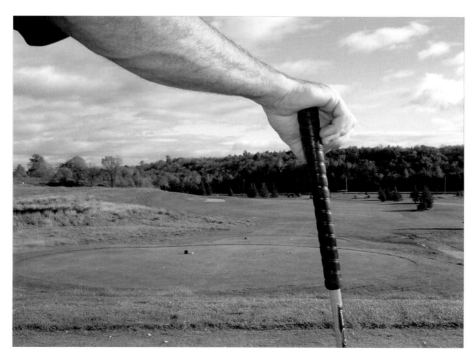

It is time for golfers to take a fresh, unobstructed look at what their actual training requirements should be.

(for wishing will not make it so), or going to the gym three to four days a week to increase one's strength and muscular endurance. For too long, training for the game of golf has been left to the domain of uninformed personal trainers who seek nothing other than more billable hours, coaching folklore that has little scientific basis, and the subtle blandishments of the commercial interests that have infiltrated all sports and, indeed, all endeavors in which peak performance is a value. Science has been all but shut out because reality is often less alluring than fantasy.

Taking quite a different approach, this book is based upon three simple touchstones:

1. Research.
2. Research.
3. More research.

You will not find a word of advice within these pages that is not supported by scientific study. This book's conclusions and recommendations will, therefore, be refreshing to some (who enjoy new discoveries that can be validated empirically) and upsetting to others (particularly those with commercial ties to certain aspects of the fitness and golfing industry), while at the same time providing ample intellectual ammunition for those who sensed that something was amiss with the training advice they have been receiving, but had lacked the data necessary to counter such claims with any type of authority.

For over ten years I have helped golfers improve their strength and their game, but more importantly, I've continued to study human physiology and the role of strength training in helping people to optimize their potential and have continued to experiment and refine what I've learned. This book is the result.

The information contained within its pages will make you considerably stronger, fitter, and will dramatically improve your game of golf in the quickest, most efficient manner presently known by science. And it will further serve as a fact-checking guide for those who truly seek to obtain the most (or Max) from their bodies and from the game that they love so much.

— John Little

1
WHERE ARE ALL THE TIGERS?

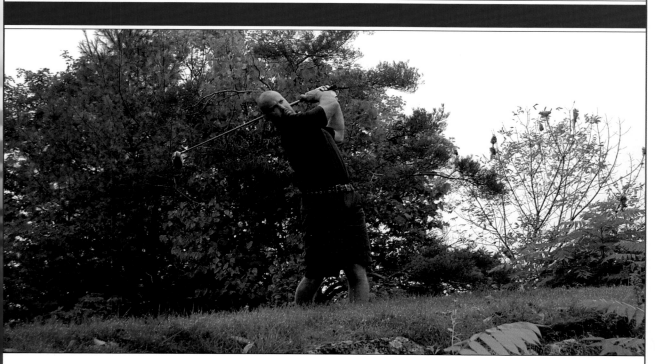

Genetics is the cardinal factor in creating an exceptional athlete.

The crowd is hushed as Tiger Woods makes his way to the tee. His swing is a picture of lithe beauty as the club arcs backwards, pauses ever so slightly at the apex of the ascent, and then changes direction seamlessly, picking up speed during the downswing. The club head connects with the ball and it rockets off from the tee, rising up seemingly into the clouds. The crowd loses sight of it until it drops down some 300 yards from where he is standing; dead center in the middle of the fairway. Another perfect drive by Tiger.

A short time later, Tiger chips onto the green from a distance of sixty feet. The ball overshoots the flag, and drops onto the green some ten feet away—but then seems to defy the laws of physics as it suddenly reverses gear and begins to roll backwards towards the cup. In what appears to be slow motion, the ball gradually zeroes in on the hole and, after an agonizing pause, drops into the cup. Tiger racks up another birdie.

"Wow!" an excited member in the crowd asks of no one in particular. "How did he do that?" Another member asks the question that most in the audience that day are only thinking: "What does it take for a person to be able to play at this level?" The answer to both questions is: ideal genetics.

Think of the greatest golfers—I mean the absolute top tier—of the past fifty years. Only a handful of names come to mind. Why? All of the golfers over the past fifty years trained for the game in exactly the same way that the greatest champions of their respective eras trained. They all worked on their swings and they relaxed. They kept their heads down and looked at the ball, they went out and bought new balls and clubs, they paid attention to the "inner game" of golf, and more recently, they have started to incorporate some form of weight training into their lives to "play more like Tiger does." So, if the majority of golfers today are all training more like Tiger does, the question remains: why aren't there more golfers like Tiger Woods walking around the local golf courses? And the answer, again, is genetics.

The fact is that somebody in Tiger Woods' family tree had spectacular hand-eye coordination, an uncanny ability to relax and focus under intense pressure, and the correct bone structure, muscle structure, and metabolic machinery to excel at the game of golf. All of these attributes were inherited by Tiger in just the right proportion which, when coupled with his almost daily neural/muscular practicing of the shots required within the game itself, allowed these traits to come to the fore and saw him blossom so spectacularly in the game of golf. This is why Tiger was on the Mike Douglas TV show at the age of two demonstrating his phenomenal aptitude for the game of golf, while you and I were refining our finger painting skills. A similar situation existed in John Daly's family tree; someone passed down the genetic factors necessary for him to be one of the greatest long ball hitters in the history of the game. (It certainly wasn't any training method he employed, since, by his own admission, he doesn't train at all!) Unless you, likewise, had ancestors that passed along such similar genetic traits, then you can adopt whatever aspect of your favorite golfer's program you want—but it simply won't make any difference; you'll never have the experience of getting sized for that Masters jacket.

You think I might be overstating the role of genetics in developing a champion? Well, consider that if you were to take a cross-section of 100,000 people, there might be 20 that possess the genetics necessary to become champions at the game of golf. Of those twenty, ten might be interested enough to take up the game, and of those ten, there might be one who would be intelligent enough to train and diet properly to fulfill his genetic potential for championship status. So the odds are 100,000-to-1 against you becoming a champion golfer. And this is why we see so few "Tigers" out on the fairways these days.

Just how big a role do genetics play in one's response to training? In a study that was conducted by M. C. Thibault and published in *Human Heredity* ("Inheritance of human muscle enzyme adaptation to isokinetic strength training." 36 (6):341–7, 1986), five sets of identical twins took part in a ten-week strength training program. The biochemical markers of strength were monitored during this time. At the conclusion of the study a wide range of response was noted between different twin sets, but the responses of the identical twin sets were, as you might have guessed, identical.

However, genetic potential—particularly for a game such as golf—is not nearly as tangible an aspect of an individual's physiology as other more measurable aspects, such as muscle length and thickness and bone structure. These are easily spotted in sports such as football, wherein the better linebackers display long torsos, short legs, wide hips, narrow shoulders and long arms, and top sprinters display short torsos, narrow hips, long legs, and a favorable ratio of the lower to the upper leg.

In golf, many of the factors that go into producing a champion are far less tangible, such as superior neuromuscular coordination, resulting in many groups of muscle fibers (motor units) contributing just the right amount of force at just the right time to result in powerful accurate drives, precision chips, and geometrically perfect putts. However, lest we forget, it is muscle in motion that that brings all of these factors together.

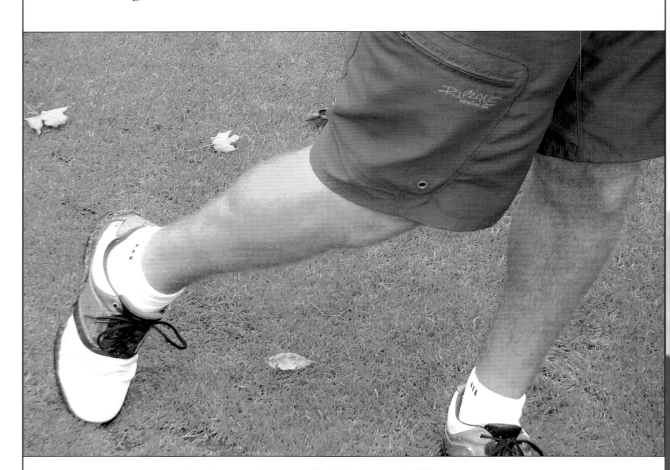

Genetic potential for excelling in the game of golf is not as easy to identify as it is in other sports.

coach, recently wrote in his introduction to my book *Max Contraction Training* that

> You can make all kinds of changes to your emotions, your relationships, but if you're physically unable to follow through on your decisions, it's all for naught. Unfortunately, one thing that I have learned, after more than a quarter of a century working with 3 million people from 80 different countries, is that most people don't truly realize how interconnected physical fitness—including strength training—is to fulfilling your potential at the highest level.

Let us, for the moment, divest the term "muscle" of its popular bodybuilding magazine and weightlifting connotations. It remains the *sine qua non* of human effectiveness on whatever plane of existence you may choose to evaluate our species. Muscle has built all the roads, cities, and machines in the world, written all the books, spoken all the words and, in fact, as Professor G. Stanley Hall wrote over 100 years ago:

> Muscles have, in fact, done everything that man has accomplished with matter. If they are underdeveloped, or grow relaxed and flabby, the dreadful chasm between good intentions and their execution is liable to appear and widen. Character might be in a sense defined as a plexus of motor habits. . . . The muscles are by weight about 43 percent of the average adult male human body. They expend a large portion of all the kinetic energy of the adult body. . . . The cortical centers for the voluntary muscles extend over most of the lateral psychic zones of the brain, so that their culture (the culture of muscles) is brain building. In a sense they are the organs of digestions. They are in a most intimate and peculiar sense the organs of the will.

Aware of the importance of muscle in human activity, virtually all of the better fitness centers today provide strength or resistance training equipment for their clients, along with advice on how to best strengthen your body. But whether or not you choose to join a fitness center or prefer to train at home with a home gym set up, it is vitally important to your total health and fitness that you engage in *some* form of muscle strengthening exercise.

So many of us rust out rather than wear out owing to a purposeful neglect of our muscles. Even those who exercise (particularly on their own) often fall far short of their full potential by neglect of proper muscle training. Many believe that they simply don't have the time for such training. After all, strength training requires at least several hours a week and a major lifestyle change, right? Wrong. Scientific research (including my own over the past two decades) has revealed that muscle size and strength—and even dramatic increases in cardiovascular

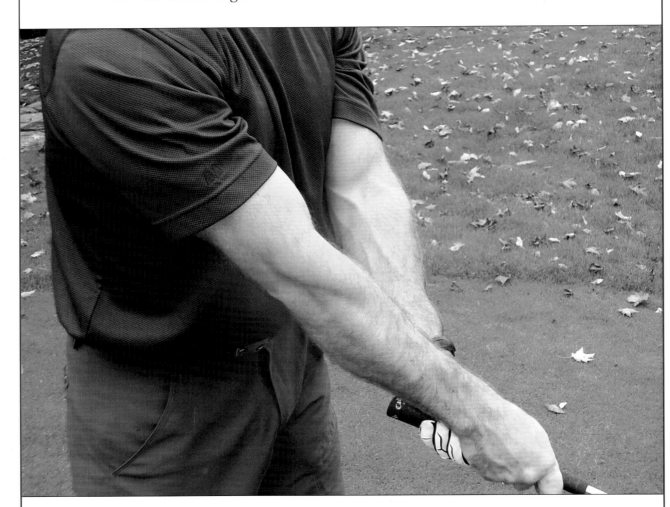

Research has clearly established that stronger muscles dramatically improve a golfer's performance.

conditioning and flexibility can be accomplished with as little as one training session per week that lasts between two and fifteen minutes. And the good news is that as you get stronger, even *less* training is required to continue to improve your level of strength fitness.

Increased muscular strength, then, will not only serve to improve your game of golf, but also your overall levels of health and fitness. With regard to golf, as the golf clubs don't move by themselves, it should be obvious that muscles are the engines that power every drive, chip, and putt. It is a rare golfer, indeed, who has the musculature of a gymnast or a ballet dancer, and yet these athletes are the models of grace and fluidity of movement. It is odd that some golfers (John Daly comes to mind) have allowed themselves to believe that training to add five pounds of extra muscle to their bodies isn't worth the effort, yet never ask how five pounds of extra fat will limit their movement—which it will.

3

A REVOUTIONARY STUDY—AND ITS IMPLICATIONS

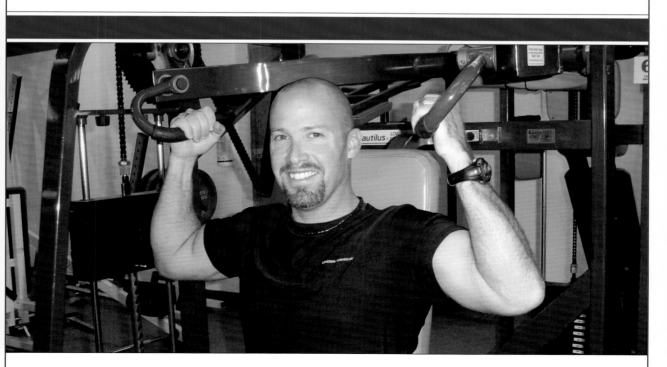

A strength training study conducted in Boise, Idaho, over 10 years ago saw golfers improve their average off the tee distance by 15 yards.

Despite all of the press in recent years devoted to the "inner game" of golf and technique issues such as how to grip the club, it is doubtful that golfers who have been golfing for many years could merely adjust their grip or mental focus and see a twenty- or thirty-yard increase in their average drive, along with a boost in overall energy and physical power. However, if you gain muscle mass and strength, the geometry of your swing will improve, not decline. This was established during a study that I oversaw in Boise, Idaho, in 1997 that produced the following documented results:

- A thirty-one-yard increase in the distance of one subject's average drive distance.
- An increase of nearly fifteen yards for the average subject of the study.
- An average increase in overall body strength of 84 percent.
- An increase in stamina, better mental focus, balance, and superior athletic performance.

And all of the golfers who participated in this study achieved the above as a result of 6.6 workouts taking an average of just 2.2 minutes of actual exercise, or 14.5 minutes of total exercise time performed over a period of six weeks. Incidentally, there were four women who took part in the study—and they actually outpaced the four men in overall strength gains; the men achieved a 73 percent gain in strength (on average) while the women achieved a 95 percent gain. In case you were wondering how the muscle groups of the whole body could be thoroughly taxed by so little training time, here is the strength increase breakdown per muscle group:

- Chest +58%
- Back +60%
- Shoulders +57%
- Frontal thighs +86%
- Rear thighs +78%
- Abdominals +170%
- Lower Back +58%
- Calves +51%

game and strength training is no exception, which is why the work-outs I advocate—and achieved such great success with—are very brief and performed very infrequently. Overtraining caused by the belief that "more is better" is worse than not engaging in strength training at all. It should be obvious, however, that golf is a muscular game; it requires muscles to swing your club, pivot your feet, rotate your hips, and arc your swing. In fact, if you are anything less than as strong as you can be, then you will be operating, by definition, at a sub-maximal standard.

When a golfer wishes to add more distance or power to his game, the answer lies in increasing the strength of the muscles he must utilize. However, for years this aspect of conditioning has all but been ignored in favor of less tangible factors. Now, however, compelling evidence is on hand to support the contention that a "stronger golfer is indeed

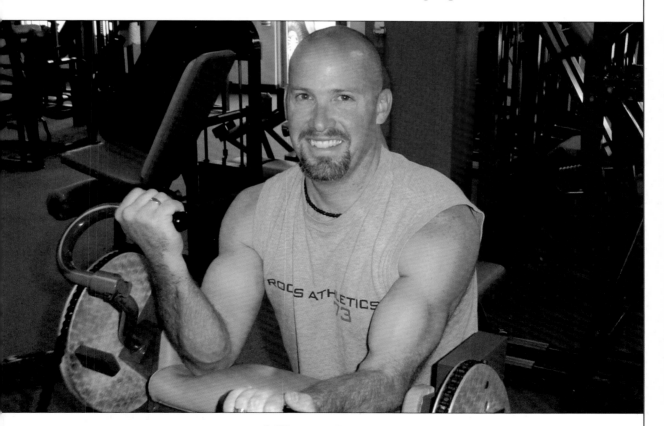

Golf is a muscular game.

a better golfer," and the good news is that it takes almost no time to become a stronger golfer.

As touched upon earlier, I know something about the particular study cited above, as I was the one who designed the training program that was employed during it, and recorded the measurements of the subjects' drive distances. However, in the years since that study was conducted, more data have been amassed to support the conclusion that infrequent workouts are most beneficial and that a particular protocol (or method of training) exists that will allow anybody to reach the upper limits of their genetic potential for strength in record time. In other words, there is a better way to become stronger, faster, than was employed during the course of the first study, and this constitutes a far more powerful technology for allowing you to become a much stronger, and much better, golfer.

4

A SECOND REVOLUTIONARY STUDY

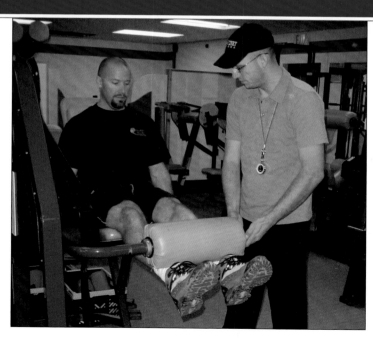

Trainer Cary Howe (right) was the lead trainer in the Nautilus North Study, overseeing each workout, recording the data, and assisting with the body composition testing.

When flipping through the pages of a golf book or magazine, there are usually a fair number of pages devoted to fitness and conditioning. None indicate when improvements will be produced from such efforts; rather the reader is told in a biblical commandment style that "Thou shalt stretch," or "Thou shalt lift weights to become stronger." Gains from following such directives, if mentioned at all, are expected to come sooner or later (and usually later), if the reader just employs these methods and keeps with the program long enough. However, gains from exercise shouldn't be a hit or miss affair. Proper training and its results are a simple matter of stimulus-response, and consequently the response (i.e., the result) should not be an unpredictable irregular phenomenon, but should (if properly applied) follow as soon as one's physiology allows.

Most golfers looking to gain strength typically lose sight of the fact that the models they are looking at in the pages of those magazines and books have been selected to model exercises solely because they are—from a physique perspective—among the genetically blessed; i.e., they have long muscle bellies and, more particularly, many more fibers packed into a given muscle than the vast majority of us. Consequently, when the physique model doubles the strength (and hence the effective cross section) of his muscles, they get much, much bigger than the average individual's whose genetics are not as strong. A champion bodybuilder, for instance, who has four times the muscle fiber density in his biceps than another individual, will, assuming both are training with sufficient intensity to double their mass, always have a muscle that is four times bigger than the average trainee's. With this in mind, the golfer must develop a more realistic perspective on what he might accomplish in terms of muscle mass increase through productive training. If one were to ask the model how he developed his muscles, the answer may be that he didn't do much of anything (remember the genetics component?). Similarly, if you ask a great golfer how he trains, his answer may yield you no benefit whatsoever (genetics again).

Many years ago, the late Arthur Jones (the founder of both Nautilus Sports/Medical Industries and the MedX Corporation) made the statement, "If you want to learn how to train a race horse, you don't ask the race horse." There is considerable merit in this statement as it has direct or preempting the growth production process. If, however, the gains showed up in twenty-four hours, then waiting two weeks could possibly delay the gains to be had from proper strength training.

In addition, if such answers could be found, then an optimal training frequency could be determined from day one of a golfer's training career, resulting in the golfer doing everything possible to maximize each of his trips to the gym and every workout he performed. And as the golfer grew stronger and moved heavier weights in his workouts, he would not be required to train as often, for it only stands to reason that the energy required for his muscles to move those heavier weights would also be greater than the energy required for him to move lighter weights, and, consequently, it would take longer to replenish a greater energy deficit than it would to replenish a deficit of lesser magnitude (i.e., lifting 100 pounds for ten repetitions does not require as much energy as lifting 400 pounds for ten repetitions). In addition, periodic adjustments could also be made at future times to determine when the training frequency would need to be modified for both the intermediate and advanced level trainee by a similar process of experimentation to determine (again) their optimal training frequency.

The entire presently "gray" area of how often a golfer needed to train could suddenly be put into very black and white terms for each individual. This thought of breaking new ground is what served as my motivation in conducting this study.

The Nautilus North Study

Presently there are so many approaches and methods of training, it is almost impossible for someone of an experimental mindset to have a control group, as there's no way that a group of subjects will not know that they are not lifting weights. For this reason, I did not have a control group for this study. The control group would be anyone who doesn't lift weights and doesn't get stronger. After all, it is safe to assume that if people don't strength train, they won't (after puberty at least) grow stronger and bigger muscles.

And then came the decision as to what type of workout the subjects should do during the study. As our subjects were not beginners (where any type of training might produce results), we opted for advanced high intensity protocols that will be discussed shortly. The training stimulus had to be intense enough that there would be a high probability that muscle growth would be stimulated. And once stimulated, it should be produced if the body was given enough time to produce it. My main focus was centered on the questions of "when" the growth would be produced and "how much" of it would be produced. As each workout should produce a positive adaptation, the job of our technicians was then to test when this adaptation manifested.

As training ought to be purposefully directed, I went to what science had to say about how to strengthen a muscle and what type of contraction was necessary to do so, and then obtained a group of subjects who were willing to submit to sophisticated body composition testing on a

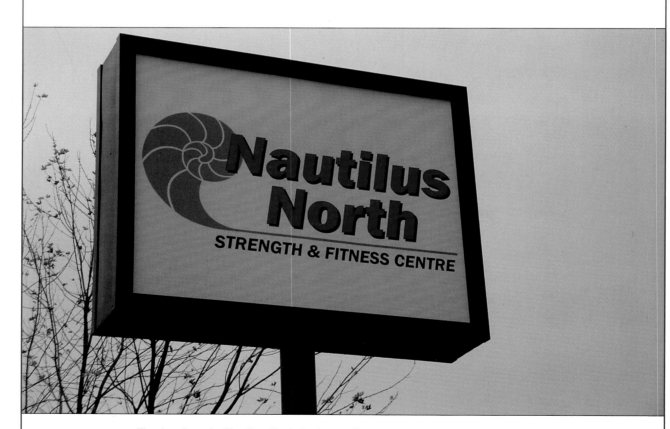

The data from the Nautilus North Study was first broken to the international public by *Ironman* magazine in 1995.

daily basis over a period of fourteen days in order to determine when the gains (however great or miniscule) would show up, thus revealing the absolute soonest one could train again without disrupting the process of recovery and growth.

With respect to how many such sets are required to produce optimal size and strength increases, the *Journal of Exercise Physiology* (online) published a most enlightening article in which, after an extensive review of all of the peer-reviewed scientific literature regarding training protocols, they concluded that one set taken to a point where an additional repetition was not possible was all that was required for building muscle size and strength in subjects with normal (i.e., non-drug enhanced) physiology.

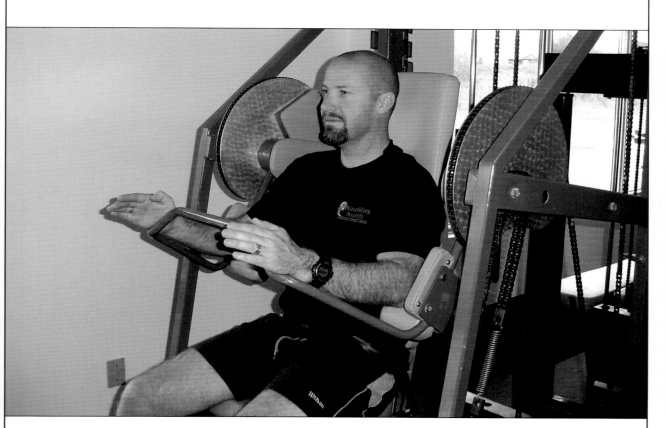

Each workout should produce a positive adaptation—if it's performed properly and sufficient time is allowed for recovery.

On a personal note, at Nautilus North Strength & Fitness Centre, which is owned and operated by my wife Terri and me, we have found by personally supervising over 42,000 workouts on a one-on-one basis that, unless an individual is grossly underweight, it is very difficult to put more muscle on him. Not impossible, only difficult. More difficult in that it requires an intensely focused effort on the part of the average trainee, and "average trainees," as a group, are not typically inclined to invest intense effort into their workouts unless they have a personal trainer who not only has a record of what they did in their previous workout (in terms of weight and repetitions) but is also able to motivate them to work out at their highest possible level. Such training is productive but not a lot of fun, with the result that most prefer to train at a modest level of intensity, two to three times per week, and precisely because their intensity is low, they don't need longer recovery periods as their weights (and correspondingly their strength levels) don't usually go up too much after their first month of training, and the stresses on the body likewise are capped. Their progress, in other words, ceases and they continue going to the gym because they believe it's "good" for them in some nebulous way or because it has become a ritual of sorts in their lives. I decided to check what would happen with clients who are very motivated to become stronger and leaner for their activities of work, sports (baseball, football, golf, and hockey), and other day-to-day existence issues. In other words, these individuals were motivated to become as strong and fit as they possibly could, thus fulfilling their genetic potential for muscular strength and size. The individuals who took part in this study were not grossly underweight or overweight, nor were they under-conditioned, being instead young-to-middle-aged-men, several of whom were fresh out of college where some ran and were coached in track and field. They were fit, quite muscular, and already very strong, but I wanted to see when the muscular gain that they stimulated from their workouts would be produced over the course of a two-week period. As the subjects would not be regaining previously held muscle mass and were already fairly well developed (regarding their individual genetic potentials for mass and strength), any gains—if they were genuine lean tissue (i.e., real muscle)—would be noteworthy and of significance to those interested in building muscle.

First, however, we needed a reliable means by which to track and assess body composition.

Enter the Body Comp Weight Analysis Center

It is very difficult for athletes and members of the general public to accurately test body composition. While it's true that there is no

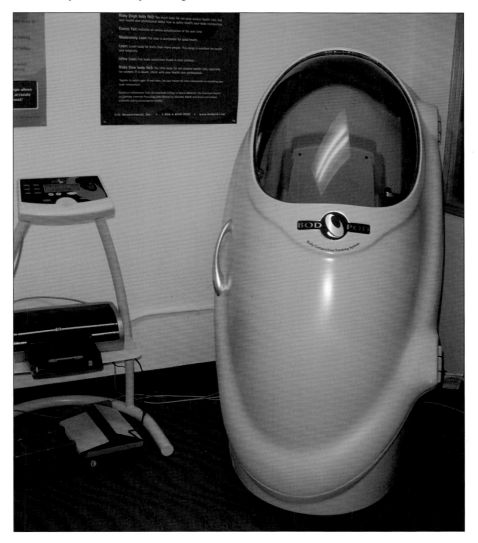

All subjects in the Nautilus North Study had their body composition tested at Body Comp, a company that employs state-of-the-art technology.

shortage of body composition testing methods available, it is also true that not all of them are accurate (some can be in error by upwards of 30 percent). Moreover, without an accurate and repeatable means of assessing body composition, you are a rudderless ship. How do you know if your training and/or diet are producing any muscle gain at all? An individual can easily gain ten pounds over the course of a month—but ten pounds of what? Water? Fat? Muscle? Fat and muscle? A body-weight scale can't determine the difference, as its sole function is to record gross bodyweight—not determine its composition. The same applies to using a tape measure (another typical fitness industry means of assessing progress); putting two inches on your arm means nothing if those two inches are fatty tissue—and a tape measure, like a body-weight scale, merely measures volume—not the composition of that volume. To make any sort of meaningful measurement relevant to determining the productivity or relative lack thereof of a given training approach, the composition of the weight and volume gained has to be accurately assessed. You need to know, in other words, that the weight you gained from training this month was as a result of an increase in the lean composition of your body rather than fat. And conversely, if you are seeking to lose fat, you need to have a reliable means by which to know if the weight you lost was fat, water, lean tissue, or a combination of all three.

Options

A Dual Energy X-Ray Absorptiometry (DEXA) machine is good for this purpose, even being sophisticated enough to measure individual limbs for compositional components down to the gram—however, DEXA uses radiation and, even though it is present in small amounts, who wants to be exposed to radiation in any form or magnitude for repeated sessions? To consistently and accurately measure body composition, repeated testing is required over a short span of time—daily in our study—in order to determine when the gains actually are produced and what the immediate effects of a proper muscle building workout are on one's muscle physiology. DEXA, while valuable for bone densitometry, which is not required to be performed so frequently, simply posed more risk than value for our purposes. Underwater weighing

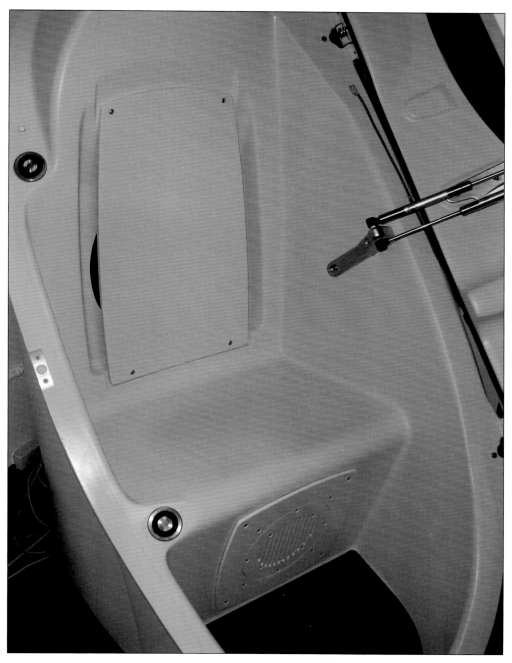

It resembles the inside of a space ship, but the Bod Pod capsule is probably the most accurate means of determining body composition on a regular basis.

(hydrostatic) is excellent and very accurate. And while hydrostatic weighing was the gold standard of body composition twenty years ago, there have been advances in composition assessment methods since that time, most notably in the areas of practicality and convenience. After all, who wanted to be dunked up to ten times for thirty seconds in an underwater tank? Moreover, I wasn't interested in having my subjects drive the hour and a half to Toronto and waiting for appointments in university physiology labs to use them. Moreover, most universities aren't interested, nor do they encourage, members of the general public to use their facilities—and certainly not as frequently as our testing required.

Bioelectric Impedance Analysis seemed promising but problems appeared with regard to both accuracy and repeatability with this technology; one client, a medical doctor in town, has a niece who is morbidly obese. He, by contrast, is a fitness freak; performing not only strength training but also competing in cross-country ski events. He is so defined that you can see virtually every muscle on his body. However, when both he and his niece tested themselves on a Bioelectrical Impedance machine, they both tested at 36 percent! Evidently, many of these machines only measure the composition of the limb or limbs in contact with their apparatus; as the current lacks strength to measure all aspects of the body. And who would want a super-charged electrical current running through their bodies, which would be required to increase the accuracy rate?

Calipers were another option, but as body fat is stored all over the body and not just in the three to four areas tested, there is no way that overall body fat can be accurately measured with such limited measurements (similarly, when body fat is lost, it comes off in a random order from all over the body and not just from the sites that the tests are conducted at). In addition, as calipers only measure subcutaneous fat deposits, their results would tell us nothing about visceral fat (or internal fat), which is the fat that typically builds up to cause serious health problems.

Moreover, of all the methods listed above, calipers have been shown to have the highest error percentage, typically the result of individuals storing fat often in different areas than those being measured at the sites the calipers target.

day-to-day affairs for the next fourteen days. To obtain a "ground zero," all of the subjects were given body composition tests prior to the workout stimulus being applied. As I was checking solely for lean (muscle) tissue increases, the subjects were not instructed to either increase or reduce their daily caloric intake. I wanted the sole variable to be the training stimulus. As a reduction in calories could compromise the lean content of the body (as if calories are restricted too low, lean tissue is often sacrificed to make up the differential), we knew that if the subjects ate their usual calorie intake (which they did) they would not sacrifice muscle tissue. This wasn't a "weight gain" study which typically sees the subjects eating more and gaining predominantly fat tissue; this was a study the sole focus of which was to determine how long it took the benefit (a bigger muscle) derived from a workout to be produced, and how much of it would be produced.

The Results of the Two-Week Study

Name	Start Lean	Finish Lean	Day of Peak Lean	Day of Lowest Lean
C. Greenfield	165.9	166.6	Day 10 (169.8)	Day 5 (160.7)
D. Craig	120.9	121.6	Day 5 (123.7)	Day 10 (118.6)
D. Beaudry	138.2	138.7	Day 1 (143.1)	Day 9 (137.8)
C. Bell	140.6	142.3	Day 6 (143)	Never went below 140.6
J. Biggs	171.9	171.5	Day 1 (173.8)	Day 4 (169)
I. Heshka	173.1	172.2	Day 7 (175.2)	Day 8 (170)
C. Howe	137.9	138.9	Day 10 (139.4)	Day 7 (135.6)
J. Little	144.5	146	Day 11 (146.7)	Day 1 (142.8)
J. Ostertag	120.9	120.1	Day 5 (122.6)	Day 1 (120.1)
T. Peake	138.4	143.2	Day 6 (147.7)	Day 9 (137.7)
J. Williams	142.4	144.1	Day 9 (145.7)	Day 3 (140.9)

Subjects were placed in the Bod Pod capsule every day for 14 days after their workout and three separate body composition tests were made. Factors such as age, gender, predicted lung volume, height, and weight were entered into the computer. After the test was completed the data indicating the percentage and poundage of lean and fat were printed out and shared with the subject to determine his optimal frequency.

Lean Gain in Two Weeks (in Pounds) Over Starting Level of Lean

Name	Start Lean	Finish Lean	Day of Peak Lean	Day of Lowest Lean
C. Greenfield	165.9	166.6 (0.7)	Day 10 (3.9)	Day 5 (−5.2)
D. Craig	120.9	121.6 (0.7)	Day 5 (2.1)	Day 10 (−2.3)
D. Beaudry	138.2	138.7 (0.5)	Day 1 (4.9)	Day 9 (−0.4)
C. Bell	140.6	142.3 (1.7)	Day 6 (2.4)	No low read
J. Biggs	171.9	171.5 (−0.4)	Day 1 (1.9)	Day 4 (−2.9)
I. Heshka	173.1	172.2 (−0.9)	Day 7 (2.1)	Day 8 (−3.1)
C. Howe	137.9	138.9 (1)	Day 10 (1.5)	Day 7 (−2.3)
J. Little	144.5	146 (1.5)	Day 11 (2.2)	Day 1 (−1.7)
J. Ostertag	120.9	120.1 (−0.8)	Day 5 (1.7)	Day 1 (same as start)
T. Peake	138.4	143.2 (4.8)	Day 6 (9.3)	Day 9 (−0.8)
J. Williams	142.4	144.1 (1.7)	Day 9 (3.3)	Day 3 (−2.5)

The above numbers indicate not body weight, but lean weight. The actual weight of the subjects—as measured by a scale—was considerably higher than indicated above, but as I was only interested in lean (or muscular) bodyweight, that is the only reading I have presented. The most striking gain was recorded by T. Peake, who produced 9.3 pounds of muscle after a mere six and a half days, and was up 4.8 pounds of muscle after two full weeks of body composition testing (all of this from only one workout). Such a rate of increase, if it could be sustained (which is very unlikely) would have seen him gain 9.6 pounds of muscle per month (and, if it was capable of being sustained into the future, 115.2 pounds of muscle per year). As this would be an unprecedented rate of increase, it is more likely that his rate of gain would arrest at some point, although we can't know in advance precisely when or what this point would be. Moreover, given that muscle will continue to respond with increases in size and strength providing it receives both the stimulus for change and the time required to produce such change, one must grant that such a gain, while heretofore unprecedented, is nevertheless possible statistically.

More likely, we should look to the *average* gain experienced by the subjects as something more realistic and therefore attainable. In

PART TWO:

THE METHOD

5

UNDERSTANDING
THE PROCESS

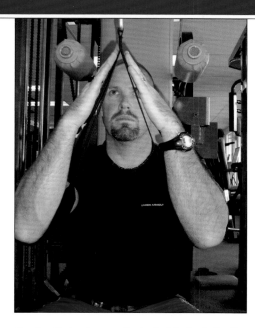

Proper exercise is a stimulus that acts upon the body. The body itself produces the response that exercise stimulates (such as an increase in muscle strength and size), and does so during the recovery period in between workouts.

I n order to better understand what a scientific training program can do for you, it might help to understand something of the process that we are attempting to engage whenever we exercise. Exercise is nothing more than a stimulus that acts upon the body. That stimulus must cause a sufficient drain of the body's (or, more specifically, the muscles') energy system to cause the body to protect itself and its energy reserves against potential future assaults of like severity by making an adaptive response. This response takes place during a period of rest that follows the application of the stimulus.

Energy is the key word in this process. We are beings that have survived periods of starvation in our history because our bodies evolved the capability to conserve energy. This ability allowed us to hang in there during lean times for a few extra weeks until we reached a different location that yielded a greater food supply (energy). Failing this, the body also cultivated an ability to diminish the size of tissues (like muscle) that require a higher calorie (energy) expenditure from the body in order to be sustained. Consequently, our genetic programming, coming down to us as it has over eons, can be simply stated like this:

OUR BODIES LIKE	OUR BODIES HATE
High Energy In	Low Energy In
Low Energy Out	High Energy Out

If we were to graph the growth and decline of human strength and lean tissue from the moment we are born until the day that we die, it would form a perfect bell curve. It would appear, metabolically speaking, that the day we are born we are shot out of a cannon, and we ride that wave until we hit the apex of our lean (muscle) and strength, which happens to fall at the very peak of the bell curve (occurring at roughly age twenty-five), followed by a gradual tapering off until it declines to the same level as our starting point. Shadowing this curve (roughly above it) would be our genetic potential for increasing our size and strength, which we would realize—if we used our muscles to 100 percent of their momentary ability during our lifetime.

Some of us may participate in vigorous athletics between the ages of sixteen and twenty-six, which would see that graph bump up a little bit (or a lot, depending upon how much of our muscles' energy reserve was called upon for the activities we performed); in which case, that graph would move proportionally a little bit closer to our genetic potential for strength and size. However, most of us (including athletes) never use our muscles at a level anywhere near 100 percent of their capacities and, consequently, nature, being an economist at heart, begins at age twenty-six to make cost cuts for energy efficiency. If, for instance, we have a fourteen-inch arm but routinely use our arm muscles at an energy output that would only justify the size and strength of a twelve-inch arm, then our arm size will be reduced accordingly. And so it goes for each muscle group of the body.

By the time most of us reach the age of forty, we have lost a great deal of our muscle mass. The result is that our resting metabolic rate has

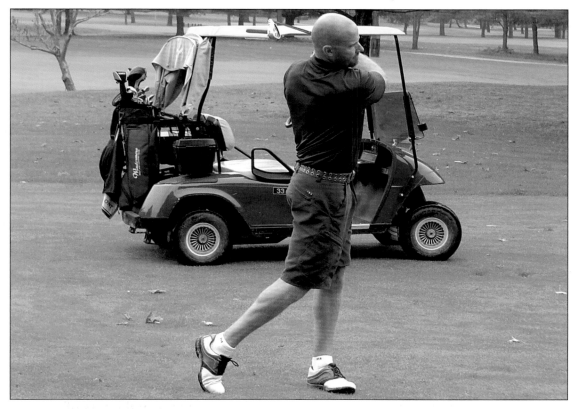

Our genetic programming is such that we will conserve energy whenever possible—such as taking a golf cart rather than walking the course.

slowed down considerably; the Kraft Dinner, pizza, and beer we lived on in college to no ill effect now seem to go directly to our midsections (or hips and thighs if you happen to be female) and activities that we used to take for granted now—should we decide to attempt them at all—leave us gasping for air and feeling like we've just climbed a very tall building with our cars on our backs. It is at age forty that most of us feel that we've "got to do *something* to get back in shape." So what do we do? We typically seek out the advice of a fitness professional—that is, someone who owns a gym. What we aren't expecting, however, is that the average fitness professional (and there are admittedly exceptions to this statement) is concerned about one thing only: turnover. That is the lifeblood of the fitness industry. The more people that will pay for a membership, the more money the individual gym owner can make and the longer he can stay in business. Toward that end, the market dictates what sells, and since getting people to work very hard and to exhaust the energy resources in their muscles is a very hard sell indeed, the fitness industry has compromised and has sold low intensity (low energy) activity as the prescription for the ailment of most people's loss of muscle and lowered metabolic rates. Given the genetic disposition of what our bodies like and dislike, the gym owners have opted for what is popular; i.e., selling the idea of going to the gym more frequently to exert small levels of energy is comfortable, and also satisfies the psychological wish of trainees to feel as though they are, in fact, doing "something" about their deteriorating physical condition. And while "something" they may be doing, it is not the required *something* that will turn that bell curve around and get them back to the level of lean that they enjoyed at age twenty-five. For this to take place requires the application of a very specific type of stimulus; i.e., one that gives the body a reason to rebuild previously held muscle—which, in turn, requires utilizing 100 percent of that muscle's energy reserves. As mentioned earlier, muscle growth, particularly new muscle growth, is a defensive reaction of the body to the stress of exercise, and the body must literally be forced to see the necessity of adding more strength and size. And as I ask the audiences at my seminars: "How do you force growth with mild exertion, light weights, and easy workouts?" And the answer is: You don't.

contract maximally while the rest of its fibers do not contract at all—
this as opposed to an entire muscle's fibers contracting all at once but
to a lesser degree. With this in mind, it stands to reason that the surest
way to involve more muscle fibers in a given contraction is to take the
muscle you're training into the one position where the maximum number of muscle fibers are capable of being activated, and a sufficient load
or resistance is applied to ensure that they are, in fact, called into play.

In a conventional set in which a weight is lifted up and down, one
starts a given movement against, literally, "zero" contraction, then moves
into a position of mild contraction, then moves into a position of greater
contraction and, finally, moves into a position of maximum contraction,
it is only this final position—the fully contracted position—that yields

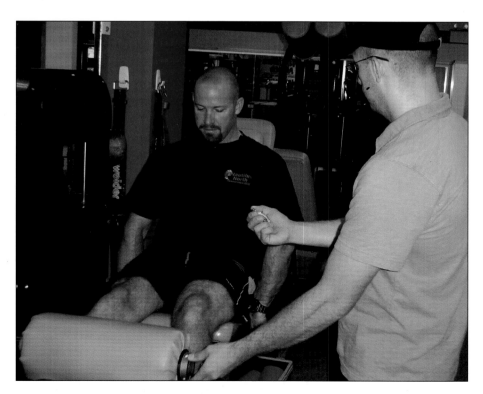

The fully contracted position of the leg extension exercise is seldom emphasized in most
conventional training protocols, and yet it is the one position where the optimal amount of
growth stimulation takes place.

the most benefit in terms of involving the most fibers. And ironically, this position is seldom—if ever—emphasized in conventional training methods.

A perfect example of this is in the leg extension exercise. Looked at physiologically, this exercise will see the trainee initiate the movement using only the barest amount of muscle fibers required to do the job. At the halfway point, a few more muscle fibers will have been called into play and then, at the position of full muscular contraction or where the legs are fully extended, as many fibers as can possibly be recruited will be activated to hold the resistance in this fully contracted position. However, long before the fibers have been stressed maximally, the resistance is typically lowered (often dropped), giving the momentarily stressed quadriceps muscles a chance to disengage (and recover to a certain extent), which is the very opposite of what you should be trying to accomplish.

This means, in effect, that in a given ten rep set performed at a typical cadence of taking two seconds to raise, one second to hold, and three seconds to lower—which lasts about sixty seconds—maximum muscular contraction takes place for a total of only six seconds. So out of a possible sixty seconds worth of maximum muscle contraction, the trainee is obtaining only one tenth of the results he is capable of deriving from the movement. Viewed in this light, it becomes painfully obvious that the trainee is wasting the other nine-tenths of the time he's been employing on the exercise. Conversely, when a given muscle group is brought into the fully contracted position and made to contract maximally against a heavy resistance for anywhere between one and sixty seconds, the maximum amount of muscle fibers and muscular energy (i.e., glycogen) that can be activated to assist in the task will be called into play until they are incapable of sustaining the maximum contraction. As soon as the trainee can no longer sustain the contraction, he will have effectively exhausted all of the muscle fibers and the energy substrates that fuel them involved in that contraction, which just so happens to be all of them.

And the sixty-second time frame is purely for purposes of illustrating the difference in efficiency between conventional or full-range training protocols and Max Contraction—or 10 percent efficiency versus roller pad. Stabilize your lower body by moving your thighs under the roller pads. Adjust the pads until your thighs are secure. Place feet firmly on platform or step and fasten the seat belt. Interlace your fingers across your waist and move your torso backward smoothly and slowly until it is in line with thighs. Sustain this fully contracted position for 30 to 60 seconds.

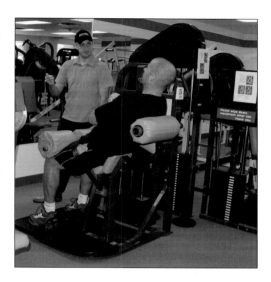

Ten Degree Chest Machine:
Lie on your back with your head higher than your hips. Place your arms under the roller pads. The pads should be in the crooks of your elbows. Move both arms (with the help of a training partner if necessary) in a rotary fashion until the roller pads touch over your chest. Sustain this fully contracted position for 30 to 60 seconds.

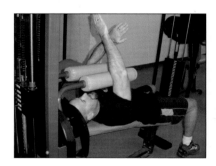

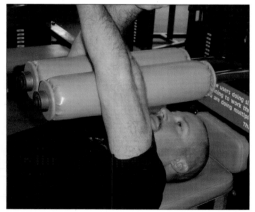

Double Shoulder (Lateral Raise):
Adjust the seat so that the shoulder joints are in line with axes of the cam. Fasten seat belt and pull hands back until knuck-les touch pads. Lead with elbows and raise both arms (again,

with the assistance of a training partner if necessary) until parallel with floor. Sustain this full contraction for between 30 and 60 seconds.

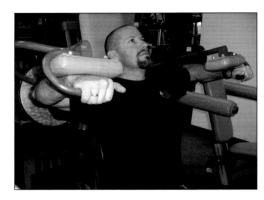

Triceps Kickbacks:
Sit down in the Super Pullover machine and adjust the seat so that the shoulder rotates on a common axis with the cam. Assume an upright position and fasten the seat belt tightly. Press foot pedal until elbow pads are about chin level (you may require a training partner's assistance) and place elbows on pads. Your hands should be hanging down at your sides and not resting on the bar. Remove legs from pedal and draw your elbows back so that your lower arms are behind the body at either side of your torso. Sustain this contraction for 30 to 60 seconds.

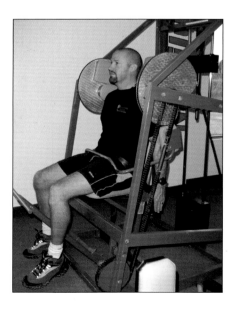

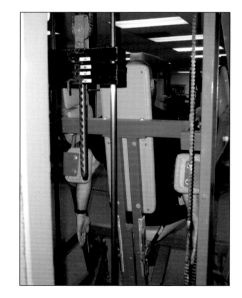

Biceps Curl:
In a seated position, place elbows on pad aligned with center of cams. Adjust seat so that shoulders are lower than elbows. Curl both arms until wrists are just in front of neck. Sustain this fully contracted position for between 30 and 60 seconds.

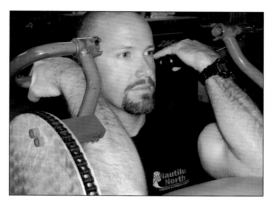

Abdominal Machine:
Assume a properly aligned position. Spread knees and sit erect. Shorten the distance between your ribcage and navel by contracting your abdominal muscles only. If necessary, have a training partner assist you into the position of full contraction of the abdominals. Do not pull with latissimus or triceps muscles. Keep legs relaxed. Sustain this fully contracted position for between 30 and 60 seconds.

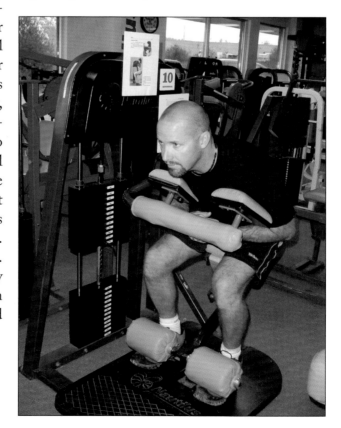

Purpose and benefits of this program

Nautilus Machine	Muscles Developed	Action of Muscles	Fitness Basis for Exercise
Hip and Back	Buttocks, lower back	Extend the spine, flexion of the spine, extend upper leg	Eliminates lower back-related problems.
Leg Extension	Quadriceps	Extend lower leg	Eliminates frontal thigh pulls
Leg Curl	Hamstrings	Extend and flex upper leg, flex lower leg	Eliminates rear thigh pulls
Calf Raise	Calves	Raise the heel	Assists in protecting the joints of the ankle and knee
Pullover	Latissimus dorsi	Move arm down and backward, stabilize torso	Eliminates lat pulls, stabilizes shoulder
Lower Back	Spinal erector muscles	Draw trunk to an upright position	Prevents lower back strain, stabilizes spine
Ten Degree Chest Pull	Chest	Draw arm across torso	Eliminate chest pulls, stabilizes shoulder
Lateral Raise	Deltoids (shoulder)	Raise, lower, and rotate shoulder	Eliminates shoulder-related problems
Multi Biceps	Biceps	Flex the arm	Assists in holding arm comfortably at proper angle
Kickbacks	Triceps	Extend the arm	Assists in holding arm comfortably at proper angle
Abdominal	Rectus abdominus	Flex spine, stabilize posture	Assists in breathing by stabilizing rib cage

Non-Nautilus Max Contraction Workout

As not everyone will have access to the same machines (Nautilus, first generation) that Tim Peake and the other trainees in the Nautilus

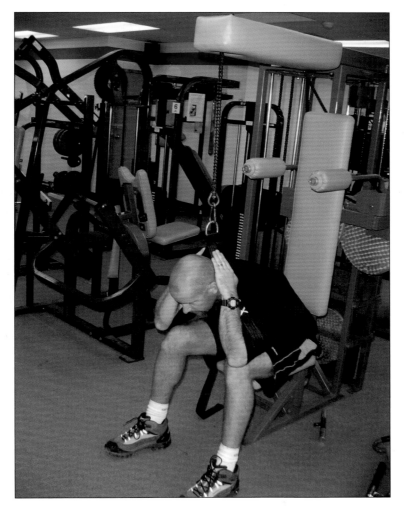

Max Strap Crunches:

Attach the Max Straps to an overhead pulley (ideally on a lat pulldown machine that has a seat and knee pad). Sit down on the seat and place your arms through the Max Straps so that the pads are over the bends in your elbows. Lower your elbows down to a point and out to the sides so that the base of the Max Straps is touching the back of your neck. Now slowly bend your torso over while drawing your elbows downwards until your elbows are almost touching your knees. Once you've hit the fully contracted position, sustain it for 30 to 60 seconds.

invaluable in this regard. Keeping a record of every proper turn (as well as every mistake—such as training too frequently) can help you avoid the pitfalls that will slow you down. A logbook serves as a record of workouts and should include daily calorie intake (including the types of foods), the weights used in each exercises, the TOC for each exercise, and the total weight lifted (TWL), which is the total weight, taken as an aggregate, of all the exercises you performed in a given workout. These figures (in particular the TWL), will allow you to know at a glance whether you are progressing in your efforts, plateauing, or even regressing—sure indicators of progress, inadequate recovery, and overtraining, respectively. By also recording your daily food consumption, you can calculate your nutritional requirements for future weight gain and loss as well as observe the effects of certain diets on moods, training drive, and progress. Experimenting with different weights, contraction times, and charting your progress can yield invaluable training data. Eventually you'll have enough information in your journal to make precise determinations.

Proceed Cautiously

If you do not have a training partner you must exercise caution when commencing any exercise using Max Contraction; i.e., lift the resistance slowly (so as not to damage any ligaments or muscle tissue) into the position of full-muscular contraction, just as you would if you were performing a regular set. However, instead of lowering the resistance, you will hold this fully contracted position for a minimum of thirty seconds and a maximum of sixty. If you can hold the resistance longer than sixty seconds, it's too light to be maximally effective and you should heavy it up by 5 percent or so for your next workout. If you can't hold the resistance for thirty seconds, then it's too heavy and you should reduce the resistance by 5 percent until you can contract the muscle against the resistance for one full second.

Training Partners

If you do train with a partner (or two) who can lift the weight into the fully contracted position for you, make sure he or she (or they) don't simply "drop" the weight into your control once you're in the fully contracted position as the sudden shock to the joint of articulation could prove traumatic. Every movement must be performed slowly, particularly the settling into the fully contracted position.

Understand the Nature of High Energy Exercise

You may notice that as your muscles fatigue they will begin to shake (sometimes rather violently) at the thirty

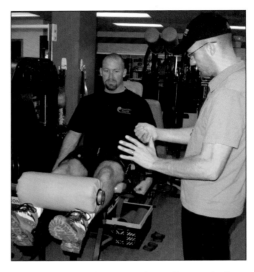

A good personal trainer who understands the physiology of the process will prove invaluable to the success of your workouts.

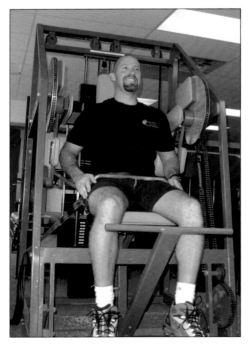

Training through a full range of motion is neither necessary nor desirable.

to sixty second mark—but this is as it should be. It's simply an indicator that your muscles are firing more and more fibers to maintain the contraction and burning up more energy. Remember, the more energy they use, the greater the growth stimulation will be. After a Max Contraction workout, you will feel like your limbs are made of jelly owing to the high volume of energy you will have expended. At which point you will be entering the stage of recovery and growth, requiring you to rest completely (i.e., take

8
ADVANCED TRAINING

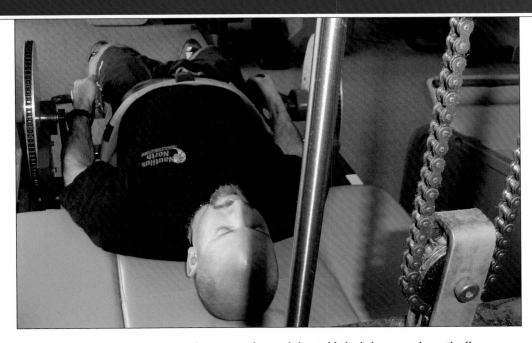

As a trainee grows stronger, the stresses he can bring to his body increase dramatically—and must be compensated for.

A s an individual grows stronger, the energy demands he places upon his body grow greater. Consider the following two workouts:

Exercise	Workout 1	Workout 2
Leg Extension	80 pounds/30 seconds	150 pounds/55 seconds
Leg Curl	50 pounds/30 seconds	90 pounds/60 seconds
Standing Calf Raise	130 pounds/30 seconds	250 pounds/50 seconds
Max Straps Pulldown	120 pounds/30 seconds	220 pounds/60 seconds
Pec Deck	50 pounds/35 seconds	130 pounds/60 seconds
Machine Lateral Raise	25 pounds/30 seconds	70 pounds/60 seconds
Flexed Arm Hang	Bodyweight (150)/ 25 seconds	Bodyweight (159) + 30 pounds/ 45 seconds
Max Straps Kickback	50 pounds/37 seconds	120 pounds/60 seconds
Crunches	60 pounds/30 seconds	110 pounds/60 seconds

These are workout charts from the same client over a three-month period. The exercises, and the sequence in which they were performed, are identical. What has changed is the amount of weight he was able to have his muscles contract against and the time that he was able to sustain those contractions. Workout 1 saw him lift a total of 715 pounds for a total of 4 minutes and 37 seconds. Workout 2 saw him lift a total of 1,299 pounds for a total of 8 minutes and 30 seconds. The energy required to lift 1,299 pounds worth of weight is obviously greater than the energy required to lift 715 pounds (by 584 pounds) and to contract against this resistance for 4 minutes and 7 seconds longer, likewise requires a greater energy output from his muscles. Consequently, the amount of time required to put back into the body the energy that he expended in getting his muscles to contract against 1,299 pounds for 8 minutes and 30 seconds will be longer than it would with any lesser amount of weight and time. In other words, your "battery" doesn't get bigger, but the drain on it from your stronger muscles gets greater and greater with every trip to the gym (or at least it should if your training is producing strength gains).

This last point is vital to grasp for the trainee who has already attained a certain level of development and strength and wishes to progress further, closer to the limits of his or her genetic potential.

What the individual will find is that he is able to drain his muscles so much more thoroughly now that he simply runs out of gas after two or three exercises. Using our illustration above, if it initially required nine exercises, 715 pounds and 4 minutes and 37 seconds of effort to drain the muscles of 100 percent of their energy, within three months of exercising once a week, this same individual is now capable of moving that same amount of weight and draining that same 100 percent of energy with only four exercises and roughly 3 minutes and 40 seconds worth of exercise.

There are two types of energy utilized by the body when producing physiological change. One is the glycogen that is stored on-site with each muscle group (and that replenishes rather quickly), and the other has been referred to as "adaptation energy," a more non-specific systemic energy, that takes a considerably longer time to replenish.

The late Dr. Hans Selye, one of the world's pioneers in stress research, was the first to label this deeper energy source "adaptation energy," and it is this energy that must be tapped or called upon for the advanced trainee to continue to make gains in strength and lean tissue mass. According to Selye, this adaptation energy is something quite apart from caloric energy, being inherited by each individual upon his birth, and its existence—and hence our adaptive (or muscle growth) capacity—is not infinite:

> Although we have no precise scientific method for measuring adaptation energy, experiments with laboratory animals offer rather convincing evidence that the capacity for adaptation is finite. Our reserves of adaptation energy could be compared to an inherited fortune from which we can make withdrawals; but there is no proof that we can also make additional deposits. We can

squander our adaptability recklessly, "burning the candle at both ends," or we can learn to make this valuable resource last long, by using it wisely and sparingly, only for things that are worthwhile and cause least distress.

As I have said, we have no objective proof that additional deposits of adaptation energy can be made beyond that inherited from our parents. Yet, everyone knows from personal experience that, after complete exhaustion by excessively stressful work during the day, a good night's sleep—and, after even more severe exhaustion, a few weeks of restful holidays—can restore our resistance and adaptability very close to what it was before. . . . If this is the case, we must distinguish between *superficial* and *deep* adaptation energy. Superficial adaptation energy is immediately available upon demand, like money in a bank account that is readily accessible by writing out a check. On the other hand, deep adaptation energy is stored away safely as a reserve, just as part of our inherited fortune may be invested in stocks and bonds, which must first be sold to replenish our checking account, thus furnishing another supply of immediately usable cash. Still, after a lifetime of constant expenditure, even our last investments will be eventually exhausted if we only spend and never earn.

And this is why as you grow stronger, and your ability to exhaust this energy grows greater, you must reduce the volume and frequency of your workouts. If you attempt to train for longer periods of time—"burning the candle at both ends," as Selye points out—then only the superficial adaptation energy is employed, but, over time, this will lead to a gradual draining of your deep reserves of adaptation energy, which could otherwise go to cover your energy debt of superficial adaptation energy. This is energy "squandered recklessly," as all of your adaptation energy will have been used up—not in the creation of stronger and bigger muscles, but in cultivating an ability to tolerate longer workouts. Use this energy "wisely" (specifically for the adaptation of size and strength) and "sparingly" (with short bursts of intense training performed infrequently). Prudent use will assure that it goes exclusively toward building larger and stronger muscles.

longer necessary (a sure sign of cardiovascular improvement) for 30 percent of the subjects who took part in the study; cholesterol medications were also found to be no longer necessary for the same 30 percent, and individuals who had been diagnosed with diabetes were found to require 70 percent less insulin—that's right, not a little less, but 70 percent less! Individuals who had come off of knee replacement surgery now found that they could literally bound up flights of stairs that otherwise had represented an insurmountable obstacle. Incredible results from a workout that lasted a fraction of the time that most individuals seeking to lose weight follow.

The reason?

In a word: science. In the past, individuals seeking to lose weight have looked to the suspect opinion of the fitness industry which exists to sell services and products, not to dispense valid scientific information (particularly when it is this simple). Consider the following medical facts:

- Muscle is metabolically expensive tissue. It requires more calories at rest than any other tissue and is responsible for 70 percent of the calories burned on a daily basis. The more you have of it, the higher your resting metabolic rate (fat burning ability) will be.
- Muscle is the first casualty on most diets and on most exercise programs. If you do not use resistance exercise, you will lose muscle. If you use resistance exercise, but it is performed for too many exercises or too often, you will—again—lose muscle tissue.
- To build muscle, it must be trained within its anaerobic pathways (up to 70 seconds). Any training beyond this point dilutes the potency of the training stimulus and could cost you muscle.
- Training too frequently prevents your body from producing or even maintaining muscle tissue.

While the above facts have been known by exercise scientists for over fifty years, they have never been applied to people's fat loss aspirations—until this program. The dramatic success of this program has resulted in it being added as a permanent part of the Nautilus North program.

A one-set workout?

During the ten-week Nautilus North/Body Comp fat loss program we recognized that the clients would have to train as intensely as they could in order to preserve (and hopefully) increase their lean tissue levels during a negative calorie balance. Doing so would lead to an increased metabolic rate and cause them to burn more calories—even while at rest—at a more rapid rate. As it is true that the greater the intensity of effort, the briefer such effort can be, we quickly recognized that some clients were "out of gas" after performing only two sets in their weekly workouts. As a result, during the course of the study we created two groups. One group was kept at three exercises (performed once a week), while the training volume of the other group was reduced to a mere two sets (performed once a week). The results? The group that did less training (the two sets once a week group), gained more muscle and lost more fat—by a two to one ratio! This wasn't an anomaly either, but rather the normal response for everyone right across the board. One of the clients in the two sets once a week group indicated that she was willing to experiment in reducing the volume of her workout even further. After the study had completed, she agreed to drop her weekly workout down from two sets to one high-intensity set per session performed but once a week. After four more weeks on a reduced calorie diet, and training on average for one minute per week, we re-tested her in the Bod Pod body composition tracking machine. We were stunned to learn that such a brief workout had resulted in her losing an additional five pounds of fat, and gaining an additional three pounds of muscle! We have since trained another dozen people in this manner, and ALL of them are outperforming (in terms of strength gains) those who are performing more sets. We will be conducting another in-depth study of this phenomenon in the near future where all of the subjects will perform one set per week and will report the findings through the Max Contraction website (www.maxcontraction.com) at that time. Certainly the implications from this would completely revolutionize the fitness industry.

We have found that in order to make judicious use of his limited energy reserves, the advanced trainee should limit himself to three exercises:

Max Strap Pulldowns

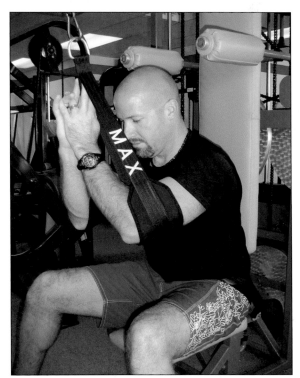

Leg Extensions

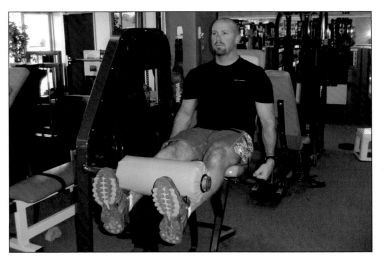

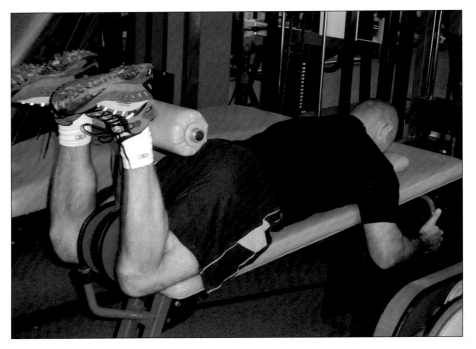

Leg Curls

These three exercises will work all of the major muscle groups in the body, and, if they feel too taxing, then reduce the workout to two exercises, either leg extensions and leg curls together in one workout and Max Strap pulldowns in the other, or Max Strap pulldowns and leg extensions in one workout, and Max Strap pulldowns and leg curls in the other.

This will keep the volume of the workouts down to a level that will allow you give 100 percent to each exercise while you still have 100 percent to give, thus ensuring that you are doing everything within your power to continue to stimulate an adaptive response to get stronger and leaner, while keeping the workouts brief and infrequent enough (they should be performed with a minimum of seven days in between, and, as you grow stronger, push that interval out to fourteen days) to allow for the adaptive response the training stimulated to be produced.

PART THREE:

ADDITIONAL CONSIDERATIONS

via an elaborate feedback system that provides information about both the environment within and outside the body. This feedback system processes information, and the brain then sends directives derived from this information to all given body parts in order to properly control all the mechanisms involved with being alive. One of the most basic characteristics of life is locomotion or movement. The importance of movement expands beyond the need to get from point A to point B; movement is essential for our species' circulatory, lymphatic, and neurological functioning. Generally speaking, in terms of our musculoskeletal system, the primary function of ligaments is to connect bone to bone, which, by definition, creates a joint. This ligament tissue expands around the joint to form a joint capsule, which provides integrity and support to the joint. Muscles function primarily to move the bones to which they are attached via movement around these joints. This is what allows our bodies to move. Muscles serve a secondary function as well, which is to support and protect the joints.

Our brain receives information about the joints and muscles via tiny nerve receptors classified as mechanoreceptors. These are situated in the joint's capsules and ligaments. It is these nerve endings that give us our kinesiological awareness (the ability to know where our body parts are as they move through space without actually having to see them). For example, close your eyes and move your hands so that they move upward in front of your face and then above your head. Now, if your nervous system is functioning properly you will know without actually seeing your hand that it is either above or below your head. It is through similar receptors that other information about a given joint is relayed to the brain. If the brain is sent information from a properly functioning joint that all is well, then the brain will send out messages to the muscles that both move and support that joint that they can remain at a relatively loose resting tonus, and that it is okay to move that joint throughout its normal range of motion. If, however, there is excessive stress being placed on a joint via some mechanism (such as heavy full-range training or even occupational stress), then the message to the brain is that "all is not well," and the brain will now increase resting muscle tonus and decrease the normal range of motion as it perceived movement of that joint as further irritation.

And this biological process is, in fact, is one way in which Max Contraction Training can increase your flexibility. As the muscles and joints are forced over time to contract against heavier weights in their strongest position of contraction, the ligaments will thicken from the compressive forces without undergoing undue shearing or stretching forces, such as those caused by full range (conventional) training practices. The increase in ligament thickness provides greater stability of the joints which reduces the need for secondary muscular support, and thus helps to produce a more flexible muscle.

In other words, Max Contraction Training will optimize your flexibility by bringing a greater degree of stability to your joints, which will afford you greater protection from injury.

If you still feel the need to warm up prior to your game, take a few easy practice swings. That—and Max Contraction Training—is all that is required.

This excess serves no useful purpose, it's potentially harmful, and it's certainly unsightly. It's what makes us overweight.

There are a number of different tables that give recommended weight ranges adjusted to height. These charts aren't of much value except to show the wide range of human variation. They don't take into consideration such individual differences as body composition (muscle weighs more than fat), skeletal size, and body type (ectomorph, mesomorph, or endomorph), all of which have an influence on weight.

The charts give arbitrary numbers and should be used only with that fact in mind, but, with or without a chart, you can tell if you're overweight. Subjectively, you know if you feel overweight and you can confirm your worst fears by looking at yourself in the mirror. Objectively, you can tell if your clothes are getting too tight and you can use the scale. If you fall outside the upper ranges of any of the height-weight charts, you are overweight.

If you are 20 percent above the recommended weight on the charts, you are probably not just overweight, but obese, a dreaded word in our society. No matter how little your food intake exceeds your energy output, you're going to put on weight. When this imbalance goes on for a time, you get overweight; if it continues, you get badly overweight; and finally, if you don't put a stop to it, you become obese.

There is evidence to indicate that obesity can also result from too little physical activity as well as just overeating. One study, using pedometers, showed that non-obese subjects were twice as active as those who were obese. And factors such as heredity, body type, stress, and anxiety can also be causes of overweight and eventual obesity.

No matter the causes, if you are heavier than your "ideal" weight (usually your weight at age twenty), you are overweight. If you are 20 percent above that weight you are obese, unless you're very muscular; and if you're 25 percent over, you are subjecting yourself to potential health problems, not the least of which is heart disease.

If you can't remember your weight at twenty (or if you were overweight then), and you can't honestly tell by looking in the mirror, then the "pinch test" is a good measure of fatness. The fat deposits under the skin (basically) reflect the total fat stored throughout the body. One of the best places to pinch is the back of the arm right behind the triceps. It's a little hard to take this measurement by yourself so you may want to ask a friend to help. With your arm hanging straight down, take hold of the skin with your thumb and forefinger at the midpoint between the elbow and the shoulder. Pull the pinched area away from the muscle. The fat will pull away with skin. If you're a man under thirty the layer of fat and skin pinched away should measure less than six-tenths of an inch; for a woman, less than 1.1 inches. If you're a man over thirty, the fold should be less than nine-tenths of an inch and for a woman, less than 1.25 inches. If the measurement is greater than it should be, you can consider yourself overweight. But don't let this scare you. It's something you need to know.

Body Composition

About 60 percent of body weight in men and 50 percent in women is water. Men have about 12 percent body fat on the average and women about 25 percent. The rest of the body (about 25 percent) is muscle, bone, blood, tissues, and organs, or "lean body mass." Muscle is heavier than fat and contains much more water (about 70 percent compared to 15 percent). Since fat contains little water, the percent of total water in an obese person is lower than in a non-obese person. The relation between total water and fat-free body weight (lean body mass) should remain constant, so when you're overweight, body composition is distorted. A combination of diet and exercise will result in the loss of fat (a large proportion of body weight), the addition of muscle, and is a very effective method of restoring the body's composition and shape.

Intensive physical training using progressive resistance machines will increase muscle mass and reduce the body's fat content. How? First, exercise with weights increases skeletal muscle size and this muscle displaces fatty tissue throughout the body. Second, strength training increases the capacity of the body's oxygen-transporting system through the cardiovascular training effect attained by the intensity of the exercise routine. It is a physiological fact that the greater the ability of the system to utilize oxygen, the greater the ability to use fat as fuel. Training increases the oxygen supply to the muscle cells so that exercise is largely performed aerobically with less lactic acid build-up. A low oxygen supply to the working muscle limits the usable fuel to carbohydrates. The less fit person produces more lactic acid which inhibits the use of fat as fuel. Conscientious weight control, along with exercise, also serves to maintain the correct balance of water and fat to muscle, bone, and other tissues.

Diet for the Golfer

Bodybuilding champion Mike Mentzer once told me of a friend of his, a competitive bodybuilder, who was so brainwashed by the health-food industry that he downed a special protein drink every two hours every day. If he didn't have this glass of magic elixir he actually got a headache and within a couple of days his ability to lift weights would decrease because he believed he was losing the protein his muscles required for strength and growth.

Bodybuilders have to be the worst offenders when it comes to believing in the magic power of foods and diet. The magic food or super pill may result in exceptional gains, provided, of course, that the bodybuilder's diet is adequate in every other way. In other words, if you're not eating right, nothing will help, and even if you are eating well, the special items are only placebos. The effects are in your head, not your body.

Of course this is nothing new. Athletes have been fanatics for centuries. The first recorded attempt to influence performance through diet occurred in Greece more than 2,500 years ago. Two athletes switched from the basic vegetarian diet of the time to a meat diet, thinking that something in the meat would replace the suspected loss of muscle during heavy workouts—just like my friend. Yet all the research done in this field is summed up by nutritionist Jean Mayer: "The concept that any well-balanced diet is all that athletes actually require for peak performance has not been superseded."

Even for competitive athletes there is no substitute for a well-balanced diet. Immediately before competition some athletes tend to eat more, but the increased energy expenditure in preparing for the events more than offsets the increased energy consumption. Research also has shown that greatly reduced or greatly increased protein consumption has no effect whatever on performance.

If a golfer is over-nourished or even adequately well nourished and yet he's not making progress, it stands to reason that his "problem" is not nutritional. If you're "over-nourished," then, by definition, you've more than covered all of your nutritional bases—so how can nutrition be a problem? If you're over-nourished or well nourished, and you aren't progressing, then your problem can only be related to training and recovery. In fact—and this is the key point—training is the first requirement, adequate rest and recovery is the second—and only then, in a distant third place, does nutrition enter the picture. And when it does factor in, it does so quite simply—all that is required in the way of nutrition for golfers is to consume a well-balanced diet, which I've already gone into some detail about. A well-balanced diet, by definition, provides the body with all the nutrients it needs. However, golfers have been subjected to thousands of pages worth of propaganda put out by the supplement companies through the various magazines over the years and thus have concluded that they *need* to supplement their diets in order to create more energy or achieve peak performance. Supplements do not build anything quicker. In fact, if you take the time to examine the small print on most supplement labels you will read the following: As with all supplements, use of this product will not promote faster or greater muscular gains. This product is however, a nutritious low-fat food supplement which, like other foods, provides nutritional support for weight training athletes.

Nutritional supplements, it should be pointed out, were developed not by golfers or for golfers but by medical researchers to provide, in fact, "supplementation" to people who through genetic or other health problems were unable to overcome nutritional deficiencies; they were never intended to be used by healthy individuals consuming well balanced diets, because medical and nutritional scientists understand what I've just revealed—that a healthy individual consuming a well balanced diet, by definition, is getting everything he needs—and the human body does not utilize nutrients beyond *need*.

Still, despite the foregoing facts, many golfers continue to feel that they require a super-abundance—and certainly more than a balanced diet would allot—of the various vitamins, minerals, and other supplements. However, I will tell you categorically that this is simply not true.

And for proof of this you need look no further than the golfing and/or fitness magazines of ten years back. For instance, if you pick up a copy of *Muscle Builder* or *Power* from the 1970s you'll read that it was milk and egg protein powder; in the 1980s it was amino acids that were *de rigeur*; in the 1990s it was MET-Rx. Presently it's creatine phosphate. In ten years, it will be something else. How scientific.

With each passing decade, the "must have" supplements from the previous decade drop from sight—so how "must have" were they? In the 1960s, for example, it was vitamin E capsules, which were being touted as wonder pills that would protect you from everything from smog and heart attacks to sexual problems. It was not uncommon then for their manufacturers to recommend up to 500 units of the vitamin E to be taken after each meal. But what is the truth about how much "E" you really need to ingest on a daily basis? For this answer, we can't look to the vitamin E supplement salesmen, but rather to independent bodies such as the Food and Nutrition Board. Going back to our example about vitamin E, we note that the RDA for this vitamin is fifteen international units daily. Thus, the "1,500 units a day" supplement (500 after each meal) actually supplies over three months worth of the RDA for this one vitamin. But ask yourself: "Is it likely that the RDA Committee is grossly in error about the amount of vitamin E needed for optimum health?" Or, putting a sharper point on it, consider the fact that our species was only able to survive and evolve by eating food that it could readily obtain. Do you honestly think that there should exist large natural barriers to our ability to access the foods needed for the maintenance of our health? I mean, it's simple common sense—to obtain the "recommended" dosage of 1,500 I.U.s of vitamin E each day our ancestors would have had to look for foods rich in "E" such as nuts, almonds being one of the best sources. To get this amount of vitamin E would require eighteen pounds of almonds a day. And wheat germ, which has also received much press as an excellent source of vitamin E, would require you to consume twenty-seven pounds of it a day in order to obtain 1,500 I.U.s. This is an extraordinary amount of food! Just one tablespoon of wheat germ weighs six grams and provides twenty-three calories. Simple mathematics reveals that twenty-seven pounds of wheat germ would require over 2,000 tablespoons a day! Which, in turn, would contain over 46,000 calories. Think about this. Is it really realistic to believe that a person can't obtain good health without either supplements or twenty-seven pounds of wheat germ? Don't be a health food fanatic—be a golfer. They're two different things.

The supplement companies respond that what the Senate Subcommittee on Nutrition recommends—the Recommended Dietary Allowances or RDAs—just aren't set high enough for good health and that the food we eat is sorely lacking in nutrients due to over-processing. Therefore, they argue, we need to supplement our diet. The truth is that the RDAs are estimated to *exceed* the requirements of most individuals, which would thereby ensure that the needs of nearly all are met. I suppose a possible exception to this rule might be in the RDA estimates of calories, or energy—but even here, obviously, it would not be a good idea to set a generous excess, since obesity is a widespread problem. The Board, for those who don't know, was assembled under the auspices of the National Academy of Science's National Research Council and is composed of large numbers of America's more respected nutritional scientists. Moreover, its membership changes periodically, both to share the burden of the work and to broaden the variety of legitimately informed opinions. The Board's Committee on Dietary Allowances is composed of subcommittees for each nutrient, or in some cases, for groups of nutrients. And it is the job of the scientists on these subcommittees to constantly reassess what is known of the nutrients, and keep up to date on the latest research reports. They also study the quantities of nutrients in the American food supply, their effects on the body, and any additional relevant information about the public's health and eating habits. Just about every five years, the Committee on Dietary Allowances publishes an updated report called *Recommended Dietary Allowances* (RDAs). This report sets out guideline recommendations for different population groups, according to height, sex, age, and weight. Thus a Recommended Dietary Allowance (RDA) for seventeen different groups of people is estimated for every nutrient about which there is sufficient data to make an informed judgment. A misperception has arisen over the years—largely promulgated by supplement companies—that the RDAs are minimums for survival, whereas in fact, they are set up to include generous safety margins. RDAs, under different names, are also set in other countries, such as Canada and Great Britain, and by United Nations agencies, and these are usually lower than the American RDAs for several nutrients. In practical terms, these committees make recommendations which should provide an excess of any given nutrient for at least 95 percent of people. Even this is very conservatively estimated, however. For example, back in their 1968 report the Committee's RDA for vitamin C for the average adult male was estimated to be sixty milligrams a day. In 1974, based on revised information, the Committee lowered this recommendation to forty-five milligrams a day—so by and large the RDAs are, if anything, overly generous, rather than inadequate. I go into the whole issue of

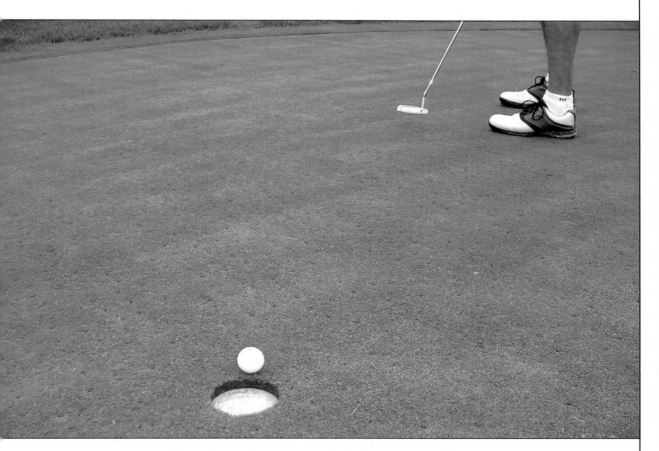

No supplement is going to turn a duffer into a scratch golfer.

nutrition and supplement fraud in my book *Max Contraction Training* in much greater detail. For now, let these few words serve as a reminder of the deceptions that abound in the world of golf regarding the issue of nutrition for peak performance. The supplement industry is reportedly an $18 billion a year business, which buys a lot of lobby power and a lot of advertising. If you're one of those golfers who have been supporting this deception by purchasing such supplements, stop wasting your money on these useless supplements and get on a Max Contraction Training schedule and a well-balanced diet. If you train hard, eat a well-balanced diet, and get adequate rest, you will be doing all that you can to improve your golf game.

aging effects on skeletal muscles to the point where they work like those found in people four decades younger.

The study was supported by the U.S. National Institute of Health, and looked at DNA expression in the muscle cells of twenty-five healthy seniors who had undergone twice-weekly resistance training for six months. It concentrated in particular on the cellular mitochondria, the "powerhouses" that fuel activity in cells. They are typically depleted in older people, with many of the genes that affect them turned on or off by age. This depletion results in a loss of muscle mass and many of the mobility restrictions often found in seniors. The lead researcher in the study, a man named Tarnopolsky, said that the genetic "fingerprints" of exercising seniors actually shifted from their age-altered state to one more closely resembling those found in young men and women in their mid twenties to thirties. "We improved or reversed to a large extent the gene signature of aging," he said. This reversal was accompanied by a 50 percent improvement in strength among seniors. He went on to state that weight training might remove some of the mitochondria damaged by age-related stresses, replacing them with genetically intact ones. As well, it may turn on genes, switched off by age, that offer muscle cells protection from damage. The seniors in the study, who had an average age of seventy, had no diseases that affected their mitochondrial function and had never participated in weight training before.

More benefits

Researchers have discovered that many of the degenerative diseases and most of the general weakness that accompanies the aging process are related to loss of muscle mass and strength. Although a certain amount of strength loss is inevitable, numerous studies—too many to be ignored—have shown that senior adults can maintain and regain muscle mass and strength at any age. Postmenopausal women, older men, and even those well into their nineties have all improved their muscular and skeleton structure and function through relatively simple programs of strength training.

The research results are remarkable: strength exercise has produced improved muscular fitness, increased bone mineral density, enhanced gastrointestinal transit, resulted in greater glucose utilization, better balance, reduced low back pain, and decreased arthritic discomfort and higher levels of self confidence and independence.

How often?

A study published by the *Journal of the American Geriatrics Society* in 1999 (47 [10]:1208–14) indicated that such gains could be obtained with only *one* workout a week—and more studies support this. A second comparison of once-weekly and twice-weekly strength training in older adults conducted by the Academic Health Care Center of the New York College of Osteopathic Medicine and the Department of Physical Therapy, at the New York Institute of Technology, School of Health Professions, Behavioral and Life Sciences, concluded that one set of exercises performed once weekly to the point of muscle fatigue improved strength as well as twice-weekly exercises in the older adult.

We have conducted our own research over the past three years at Nautilus North, most of which has been published, and we've seen incredible results from as little as two minutes of strength training performed once every seven to ten days. Results such as significant reductions in blood pressure and cholesterol levels, diabetics being able to reduce their nightly insulin intake by up to 70 percent, and strength and mobility improving from having to get around with two canes and only being able to leg press 60 pounds, to not needing canes and being able to leg press in excess of 800 pounds!

How high is up?

Doug McGuff, M.D., who owns and operates Ultimate Exercise in South Carolina (www.ultimate-exercise.com) has a client that trains once a week with three exercises and has been doing so for seven years. This man performs a pulling exercise (seated row) with 280 pounds, bench presses 320 pounds and leg presses 600 pounds—and he's ninety-three years old!

The Anti-Aging Prescription

There are ten bio-markers of aging:

1. Bone density: Because calcium tends to be lost from the bones when people age, it makes the skeleton weaker, less dense and more brittle, which typically leads to osteoporosis.

2. Body temperature regulation: The body is supposed to maintain an internal temperature of 98.6 degrees, but as people grow older they tend to lose muscle and the heat that muscle provides, thus becoming more vulnerable in their body temperature to hot and cold, which often leads to illness.

3. Basal metabolic rate: Our rate of energizing or determining how many calories our bodies require to sustain their internal processes, declines by 2 percent per decade after the age of twenty.

4. Blood sugar tolerance: The body's ability to use glucose in the blood stream declines with age, thereby raising the risk for type 2 diabetes, which is one of the fastest growing spreading diseases in the country.

5. A decline in muscle strength: Older people are less strong because of the gradual deterioration of the muscles and motor nerves, which begins at the age of thirty for most people.

6. The fat content of the body: Between the ages of twenty and sixty-five, the average person doubles his ratio of fat to muscle. This process is exacerbated by a sedentary lifestyle and over eating. Exercise can often serve to retard appetite and, conversely, when you're not training, you tend to be more hungry—and to eat more often.

7. Aerobic capacity: By the age of sixty-five the body's ability to use oxygen efficiently declines by 30 to 40 percent.

8. Cholesterol and HDL ratios: Around age fifty HDL (or "High Density Lipoproteins," the so-called "good" cholesterol that protects the body against heart disease) loses ground to the LDL (or "Low Density Lipoproteins," the so-called "bad" cholesterol); a phenomenon that dramatically increases the risk of heart attack.

9. A decline in muscle mass: The average American loses 6.6 pounds of muscle with each decade after young adulthood and the rate of loss increases after the age of forty-five (but only if you don't do anything to replace it).

10. Blood pressure: The majority of Americans show a steady increase of blood pressure with each decade of age.

And the one and only activity that's been proven scientifically to affect all ten of these bio-markers of aging is strength training. No other activity comes close not even aerobics! And Max Contraction is the most efficient form of strength training available.

If you're a senior citizen and you haven't strength trained—start. Your quality of life will increase enormously.

import of the "mind" in golf. Sure, the mind is important. Without it you couldn't even tie your shoes let alone engage in swinging a golf club, but the mind is not nearly as omnipotent as some "authorities" would have you believe.

The mind is important in keeping you motivated to get into the gym and train intensely enough to stimulate your muscles to grow stronger—which, as I have discussed in previous chapters—is not an easy task (particularly as you grow stronger and the energy drain you face each workout grows greater). In fact, it's downright uncomfortable. So much so, in fact, that anyone who feels the inclination to engage in "visualization" or cognitive gymnastics really isn't training—they're simply going through the motions and relaxing, because relaxation or "sleep" is the time we are best able to engage in such flights of fancy (we just refer to them as dreams).

Q: You're correct that training to the max is difficult. How do you stay motivated to give 100 percent of your energy to the task of working out year after year?

A: The ethos of Max Contraction Training is: be willing to give 100 percent of what you have to a given task. It is the cornerstone of my personal philosophy, and those of others who have likewise embraced this method of training. Stated another way, the concept is that if you are going to attempt anything, then give it everything you've got—or don't bother. Nobody in life benefits from a half-assed effort: not in work (employer and employee), not in love (where neither party has a maximum emotional investment), and certainly not in exercise (which must be intense enough to stimulate an adaptive response). When we are able to transcend, if only by a degree, our previous levels of effort and energy output, we invariably make quantum leaps in progress. These Max efforts help us break through to higher functional levels, and, as a result, they are powerful learning experiences that teach us much about our physical and intellectual potential.

According to psychologist William James, "Compared with what we ought to be, we are only half awake. Our fires are damped, our drafts are checked. We are making use of only a small part of our possible mental and physical resources." All of us, in other words, operate well within our existing limits, failing—as William James might say—to make full use of the power we know we possess. Our day-to-day existence is typified by this reluctance to engage in an all-out physical effort; it's something that is ordinarily avoided when possible. As mentioned earlier, we are a species that has survived owing to a cultivated ability to conserve—rather than expend—energy. Consequently, other than in athletic competition, such effort is produced typically in emergency situations only. Only a person fired by a strong, almost overwhelming sense of purpose and meaning will be able to train his muscles to the point where he has tapped all of their energy.

So, the question becomes: how strong is the value you place on getting stronger? On getting leaner? On becoming a better golfer? If it's not that strong, then the reality is that you will not be able to moti-

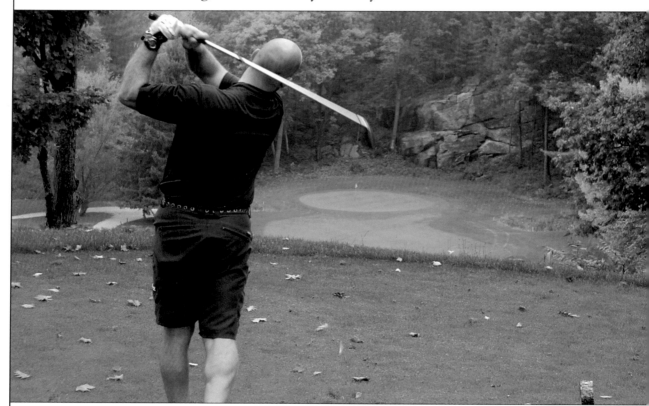

Seeing constant improvement in your strength (and its positive effects on your golf game) will often serve as sufficient motivational fuel to ensure that you continue to give your all to each workout you perform.

that was training two times a week, was cut back to one time a week. And in doing so the experimenters noted that the subjects' rate of progress improved. And there have been other similar studies; this has been duplicated in other studies in different age subjects wherein the experimenters take them and decrease their training frequency and find that they actually do better—particularly the elderly. But even in younger subjects this is borne out. Regarding seniors, the Academic Health Care Center of the New York College of Osteopathic Medicine and the Department of Physical Therapy, New York Institute of Technology, School of Health Professions, Behavioral and Life Sciences, published a study comparing the results of seniors training once a week and seniors training twice a week, and found, in their words, "no difference in strength changes between training once a week versus twice a week after 9 weeks. . . . One set of exercises performed once weekly to muscle fatigue improved strength as well as twice a week in the older adult." There are more data coming in each year to support the fact that training more than once a week represents nothing more than more time needlessly spent in a gym.

For instance, the May 1993 edition of the *Journal of Physiology* contained a report about a group of men and women aged twenty-two to thirty-two who took part in an exercise experiment in which they trained only their biceps muscles in a negative-only fashion to a point of muscular failure. Negative or eccentric contractions (which consist of lowering—rather than raising or lifting—the resistance) are considered by some exercise physiologists to be more intense than positive or concentric contractions because of the fact that more weight can be employed and, thus, the intensity of the exercise can be increased. All of the test subjects were found to be most sore two days after exercising (a common occurrence by the way) but the soreness in their biceps was gone by the ninth day. However, what was even more telling was not the highly subjective report of "soreness" in the muscles, but the far more tangible report of the impact of the workout on their strength levels. The day after the exercise the subjects exhibited what the experimenters termed "a dramatic 35% loss of strength. . . . even on the tenth post-exercise day the muscles had recovered only to about 70% of their control strength."

The experimenters, John N. Howell, Gary Chleboun, and Robert Conaster (from the Somatic Dysfunction Research Laboratory of the College of Osteopathic Medicine and the Department of Biological Sciences at Ohio University, Athens) concluded in their summary that "muscle strength declined by almost 40% after the exercise and recovery was only slight 10 days later; the half-time of recovery appeared to be as long as 5–6 weeks."

Given that a muscle must recover before it overcompensates or adapts, the positive change a trainee is seeking from exercise will only arrive after full recovery has taken place, meaning that many weeks "off" from training will be required before the benefit (the adaptation from the workout) can be produced. And lest you think that overtraining is of concern only to those who engage in heavy strength training, additional research conducted on marathon runners (who engage in highly repetitive, lower intensity activity) by Michael Sherman at Ball State University in Indiana also indicated that the recovery period required after even low intensity (high volume) training can extend to a period running into months. In the January 1985 issue of *American Health* magazine, Stephen Kiesling reported that "Sherman found that even after a full week of rest, marathon runners had not regained pre-race strength and power. Returning to [even] moderate running after the marathon delayed recovery. And some races may take months to recover from."

It is also worth pointing out that the iconic runner Roger Bannister revealed in the December 1996 edition of *Runner's World* magazine that he in fact *rested for five full days* prior to his breaking the four-minute mile barrier. Bannister believed that *not* running during those days prior to the race allowed him to take his mind off the competition, but from the research cited above, his days of rest actually allowed his body additional time to recover from his running sessions and his recuperative subsystems to replenish and grow stronger, thus allowing him to run the first-ever sub-four-minute mile.

In seriously considering the data cited above, we are forced to conclude that the recovery process can take not one to two weeks, but quite possibly up to ten to twelve weeks! That is to say, up to three months off might be required in order to simply recover from an intense workout.

The conclusion to draw from the data cited above (as well as what I indicated in previous chapters) is simply that training—of almost any variety—creates far greater demands on the body's recuperative subsystems than most people (including many strength coaches and personal trainers) realize. Muscular adaptation is a biological process, and therefore it is not mediated by traditional societal considerations such as the Gregorian calendar with its seven-day week. Adding additional muscle to your body and improving your fitness level is not an easy process (if it were, there would be a lot more fit and muscular—and a lot less overweight—people running about the fairways), with the result that you cannot force your body to become fitter and stronger by subjecting it to marathon-style low intensity training (mild exertion) sessions. As your body can already handle this level of intensity, there is no reason for it to alter its present level of fitness and strength. Your objective in training—whether it is to lose fat, tone up, strengthen your muscles, protect your joints and connective tissues to enhance mobility or athletic performance, or simply to look better—will never be realized by training geared to seeing how much exercise you can tolerate, nor how many different exercise sessions you can squeeze into a seven-day period.

Like medicine, exercise must be applied in the correct dose and the correct frequency in order to produce the optimal response from your body. Any more than the precise amount required will result in your body "overdosing" on the stimulus, which can take many months to recover from. When it comes to exercise, "more" isn't better. Any amount more than the least amount required to realize your objectives is overtraining, by definition.

In conclusion, then, it would appear that the best exercise one could perform—no matter what one's personal choice in exercise—is the exercise of restraint.

Q: If I grow stronger, can't I perform more exercise? I'm not clear on how a more advanced trainee can benefit from performing less exercise. Please explain.

A: Bear in mind that as an individual grows bigger and stronger, his or her energy output increases proportionally, as the heavier the resistance that the muscles are made to contract against, the greater the energy output that is required to perform these heavier contractions, and the longer it takes these energy reserves of the human body to replenish themselves. Golfers who ignore or otherwise fail to make their peace with this biological law will soon see their strength training progress grind to a halt. The only way such plateaus or sticking points can be obviated is if the golfer continues to make the requisite adjustment (in the form of adding additional "rest" or "recovery" days into his training schedule) to compensate for the increasing demands of the training stress to which he is subjecting his system.

The reason being that each time an individual becomes stronger, he has increased the intensity of his workout, and each time the intensity of his workout is increased, the longer it takes the body to put back what was used up (and more time must be allotted for overcompensation—the

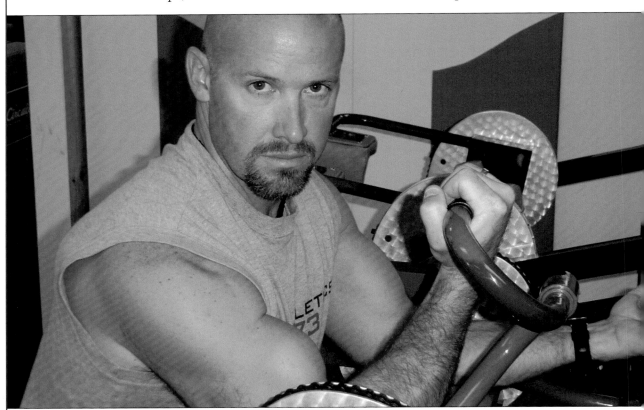

As you grow stronger, you simply use up more energy more quickly. You don't, however, replenish your energy reserves quicker. Consequently, as you grow stronger you need to train less frequently.

strength gain—to take place). Additionally, each time one increases the intensity of one's workout, a corresponding adjustment must be made to the volume of his effort during the workout. For the same reason that an all-out sprint is more intense than a walk, it cannot be continued for as long a period of time (i.e., you can walk for miles but only sprint for a handful of yards). The same is true with strength training exercise; i.e., the more intense the workout, the shorter its duration has to be.

When one is a beginner, the stress one is capable of generating and thus subjecting one's muscles to is minimal, with the result that one has the luxury of being able to endure repeated exposure to such a low intensity training stress (e.g., training with many sets, many days per week, and many routines, if one so desires) and will make progress—perhaps not as significant progress as he would make if he trained more intensely, but then again, a twelve-inch arm contracting maximally does not place the same demands on the body's energy systems as does a fifteen-inch arm contracting maximally. A beginner's muscles are literally too "weak" to generate the intensity required to thoroughly tax the body's energy systems so as to prevent recovery from occurring between training sessions. However, as the beginner becomes stronger, his energy output and ability to raise the stress he can subject his muscles to increases (in some instances quite dramatically), with the result that he quickly finds that he can no longer recover and grow stronger in twenty-four hours, forty-eight hours, seventy-two hours— or even longer. It is at this juncture in his training career that the trainee should begin to insert additional "off" or "rest" days into his routine and to reduce the duration of his exposure to the training stress.

This last point is one of the most crucially important elements of exercise science, and has been completely overlooked by almost everyone. With very few exceptions, almost every personal trainer has his clients stay on the same volume and frequency protocol virtually forever. Once the fundamental principles are understood, however, the issue of progressively decreasing the volume and, especially, the frequency of one's training becomes the most pressing issue. If the trainee bears this in mind, he will never reach a sticking point, there will be no need to engage in such protocols as "periodization" (wherein you train efficiently, i.e., intensely, for certain periods of time and then train inefficiently, i.e., with less intensity, for other periods), and he will actualize his full strength and muscular potential in a relatively short time.

Q: Do you think that it's a good idea to do a little bit more abdominal work—to really strengthen the "core" muscles better? I believe that they contribute to trunk rotation, which would be helpful in golf.

A: The so-called "core" muscles are the abdominals. And as the function of the abdominal muscles is to draw the trunk toward the thighs, this action is perfectly covered with the Max Crunch exercise using Max Straps. Once you've drained the energy out of the abdominal muscles in this fashion, there is nothing else, in terms of exercise, that is required to strengthen them. It must be remembered that the abdominals are skeletal muscles—just like the biceps and calves—and, therefore, their training requirement is no different from these other muscle groups. The abdominals don't require volume training but rather high-intensity training, which, as we know, must be intense, brief, and infrequent. Training your muscles in this manner will result in superb abdominal strength. Rely on practicing your swing to perfect your technique. Incidentally, trunk rotation is actually a function of the oblique muscles and the hips, with the abdominals contributing very little to the action.

Q: I recently bought your audio lectures and read your book—terrific information. However, I did not see anywhere what you recommend for preparation, such as warm ups, stretching out, etc. It would seem unreasonable to come into the gym and start lifting a max weight without some sort of warm up?

A: Warm ups are very important, but also a very individual-oriented phenomenon, depending on such things as the individual's age, existing physical condition, prior training history, and injury history. For these reasons, it is difficult for anyone to prescribe such a program without dealing with each trainee on an individual basis. Typically warm ups are required for full-range or conventional training, as you are moving a weight throughout a full range of motion and, as the weights get heavier (for your working set), the potential shear forces on joints and connective tissue increases. As Max Contraction is motionless exercise, and the exercise that is performed is executed in your strongest range of motion (i.e., where your leverage is optimal and your muscles, joints, and connective tissues are strongest and, thus, best able to accommodate it),

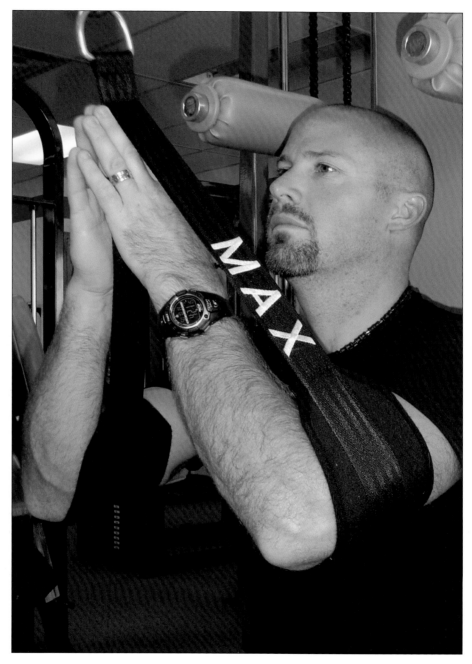

Max Straps provide direct resistance to the muscle being worked (in this instance, the latissimus dorsi muscles of the upper back), resulting in a greater degree of growth stimulation.

group you are attempting to train. Max Straps do this very efficiently and so are featured in the book and training DVD for that reason. For those bodybuilders who wish to learn more about Max Straps, please visit Max Contraction online at www.maxcontraction.com.

Q: It is widely known that strength increases as the result of isometrics are joint angle specific, in that the strength increases only occur at the angle the contraction was held at. In your book you suggest taking a joint to the end of its range of motion so that the muscle is in a fully contracted position, and then applying isometric tension at this point. My question is, will this method allow uniform strength to be gained throughout the full range of motion, or will it still be restricted to the joint angle, in your case at the end of the range of motion?

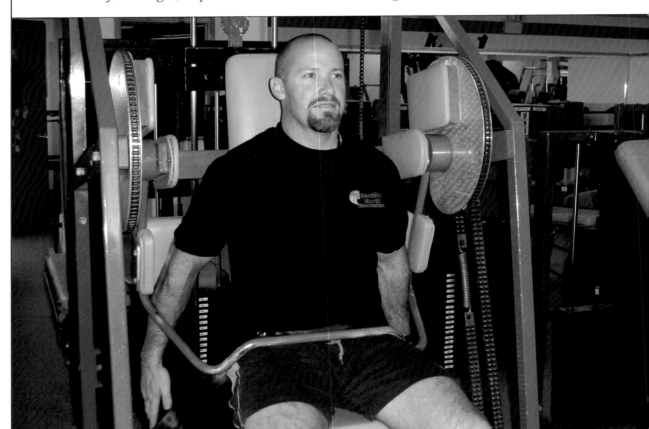

Full contraction—not full range—is the most important factor for strengthening muscles.

A: I, too, have heard about the alleged "non-transference" of strength increases in one's strongest range to one's full range. I believe Arthur Jones even conducted some testing in the 1980s on this, but that he found that only *some* (whom he dubbed to be type "S" or "specific") did not record a transference of strength from one position of flexion to full range. Others, whom he classified as type "G" (for "general") did record a positive transfer to full range strength after training exclusively—and statically—in one position. However, my answer to your question would be in two parts.

First, the primary factor in muscle fiber recruitment and, thus, muscle fiber stimulation, is the intensity of the contraction of a given muscle. That is, how heavy the load is that your muscles are made to contract against, with the heavier load requiring more fibers to accomplish the task of contraction. It used to be believed that if you trained a muscle "through a full range of motion" you would be "training the full muscle," whereas if you "trained a muscle in one position, you would only be developing one part of the muscle," when actually the reverse is true; i.e., if you train through a full range of motion, then you will only develop part of the muscle, predominantly slow twitch and intermediate twitch fibers, as those are the only fibers that can be recruited owing to the fact that a full range of motion restricts you to using a lighter weight than what you are actually capable of maximally contracting against. As muscle fibers are recruited solely by the amount of force they must produce (i.e., the amount of weight they are made to contract against), and as you are capable of contracting against more weight in the fully contracted position than you are restricted to using in your weakest range of motion, you will recruit and therefore stimulate all fibers (i.e., the full muscle) with a Max Contraction set.

Muscles contract by shortening or reducing their length, therefore the one position where all of the fibers are contracted would be (by definition) the "fully contracted position" (what I term the position of "Max Contraction"). In other words, the two factors responsible for maximal stimulation of a given muscle both involve "maximums"; i.e., that the muscle be in a maximally contracted position and that the load imposed on the muscle while in this position be the maximum that the muscle is capable of contracting against. This said, what fibers would not be recruited from this protocol? If all the fibers are recruited as a result of the two requisites indicated, then that would include the fibers involved during the first sixteenth of contraction, the first quarter of contraction, the first third of contraction, the first half of contraction, the third quarter of contraction, and so on—as all of these same fibers are involved in the shortening or "contracting" process. As a result, all fibers that can be stimulated to grow stronger will have been stimulated to grow stronger from a "zero" range of motion—providing this zero range of motion takes place in the muscle's fully contracted position. Jones, to my knowledge, tested his subjects at different points in the range of motion and, as the fully contracted position is the only position where all of the fibers are brought together and where, indeed, the contraction can only be said to be truly "maximal," it is not surprising that a weak range contraction would produce results only proportionate to the amount of fibers recruited and stimulated in that range. Any other point but that of maximum contraction is by definition a sub-maximum contraction, and hence less productive. I would also mention that Peter Sisco conducted an informal study with motionless (static) exercise and determined that there was a 35 percent transference of strength to full range or dynamic strength. It might be argued that 35 percent proves that a full transference of strength did not take place, but when you consider that none of these trainees on the study had gained any strength using full-range of motion exercise for several months prior to performing the static holds, a 35 percent increase in their full-range positive strength is considerable. Second, I don't believe an increase in full range of motion strength to be the benchmark that many others believe it to be. If you increase your strength in a given position by 80 percent, and you gain seventeen pounds of muscle in the process, you would obviously be accomplishing your objective of building a bigger, stronger body. The fact that this can be accomplished in so little time (seconds a week versus the hours a week required by conventional approaches) means that this is a more efficient means of achieving your objective. And unless you absolutely require the ability to bench press throughout a full range of motion many hundreds of pounds on a progressive basis, what would be the point of devoting hours and years to the cultivation of this talent? You don't need to do this to become bigger and stronger; indeed, it is actually an impediment to becoming bigger and stronger as a full range of motion actually reduces the amount of resistance your muscles are capable of contracting maximally against, thus providing sub-maximal overload (and results) to your muscles. Training throughout a full range of motion does NOT (again, contrary to the popular view) enhance flexibility (which has a strong genetically mediated limit to begin with; i.e., a muscle cannot "increase" its flexibility without either tearing something or losing its tonus) more thoroughly than performing a Max Contraction (as the stronger the muscle—the whole muscle—the more secure the joint and mechano-receptor sites responsible for tonus/tension and relaxation or stretch). Indeed, there is ample evidence that training with moderately heavy weights throughout a full range of motion will actually increase your chance of injury owing the sheer forces that impinge on joints and connective tissue when bones and ligaments are required to move through arcs and positions of disadvantaged leverage.

If your objective in training is to have a stronger full range of motion (that is, to be able to lift heavier weights through a full range of motion), the best approach would be to train specifically for this skill—by performing only full range movements. This will, however, severely compromise your ability to build maximum size and strength in your muscles as, again, your muscles are capable of contracting against much heavier weights than a full range of motion allows you to employ. And the heavier the weights, the more intense the contraction, and the more intense the contraction (when combined with proper rest periods), the greater the muscle growth production.

Q: Muscle fibers don't usually run the length of a muscle. So if you only build the fibers in an isolated part of the muscle, you don't build all the fibers above and below it. And that just has to limit your muscle growth, right? This is one law of exercise physiology you can't sidestep.

A: I won't sidestep it, but meet it head on. This is a specious argument because motor units distribute their fibers homogeneously throughout the length of a muscle. So when you recruit motor units, you do so homogeneously throughout the whole distribution of the muscle. The nerves that enter a given muscle divide out into threads that resemble branches on a tree. Each branch ends at the muscle cell and carries the electrochemical current that causes each muscle cell to contract. When

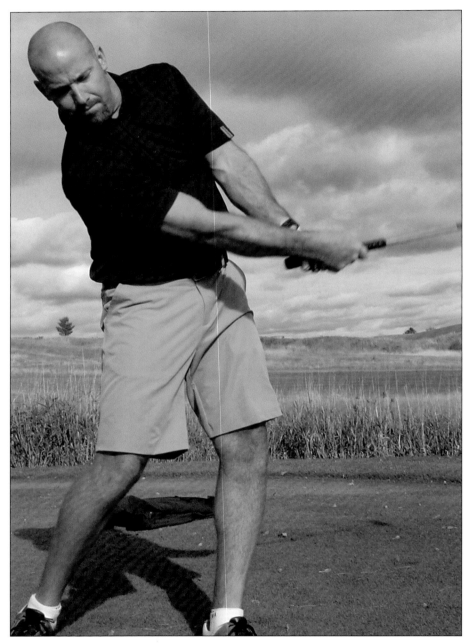

The notion that training with Max Contraction will only develop the muscle and strength and size in the range in which the contraction is performed is specious because motor units (groups of muscle fibers) distribute their fibers homogenously throughout the entire length of a muscle.

this current is released, all of the cells serviced by the branch (a single neuron) contract simultaneously (the all-or-none law of muscle fiber contraction), not some to the exclusion of others. It's simply not possible to isolate one portion, border, or ridge of a muscle. But don't take my word for it. Consider this excerpt from Dr. Fred Hatfield's book on *Bodybuilding: A Scientific Approach*:

> The cells associated with each motor unit are spread all through the gross muscle; all portions of the gross muscle are affected similarly by a given exercise and therefore develop similarly. This is called the principle of noncontiguous innervation. Using many variations of an exercise for one muscle in no way ensures more growth or different growth patterning than does performing the basic exercise. . . . The shape of that muscle will not be affected by variations in the angle or position of stress application. Does this mean that all a bodybuilder has to do is perform the basic movement and rid himself or herself of the array of supplemental exercises for a given muscle? I suspect it does.

Q: Were the subjects in the Nautilus North study regaining previously held muscle mass?

A: No. The subjects who took part in the Nautilus North study had been training steadily for a period of at least six months with high intensity protocols and had been training only once a week in this fashion prior to the study. None of them were regaining previously held muscle mass but were hopeful to build new muscle mass. The subjects in the Nautilus North study were not grossly underweight or overweight, nor were they under-conditioned, being instead young to middle-aged men, several of whom were fresh out of college where they ran track and participated in activities such as football, hockey, and martial arts. They were not previously over-trained and then able to take advantage of the two week testing period for recovery, and they were not made to drink lots of water before testing or to eat any particular diet beyond what they normally consumed on a daily basis and had been consuming for the previous several months prior to the study being conducted. These were simply fit, and, in some cases, already very strong individuals who had an

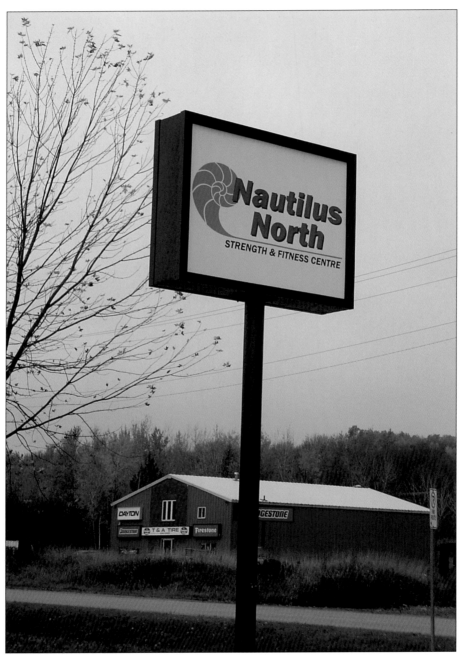

The subjects who took part in the Nautilus North Study were building new muscle mass, rather than regaining previously held muscle mass.

interest in seeing what effect a high intensity workout had on the body and what if any gains could be produced from a solitary workout. As the subjects would not be regaining previously held muscle mass and were already fairly well developed regarding their individual genetic potential for mass and strength, any gains were noteworthy and of significance to those interested in building new muscle from exercise.

Q: I'm still not clear on the whole issue of recovery ability. Are you saying that everyone now only needs to train once a week?

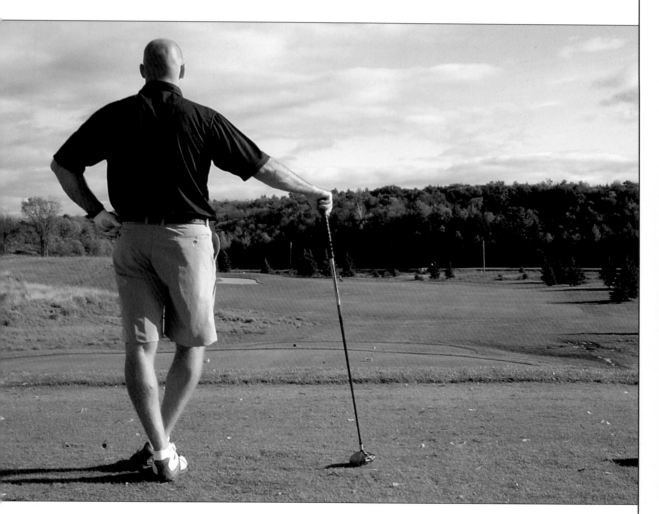

Golf as often as you wish—strength train as little as is required.

A: What I'm saying is that as you get stronger, you will need to train less frequently. You might think of it this way: When a beginner works out it takes "X" units of time to recover from the workout, an intermediate trainee with his greater energy expenditure will require "Y" units of time, and the advanced trainee requires "Z" units of time. We should get out of the rut of thinking in terms of seven-day periods—particularly in matters pertaining to human biology. The body simply requires the amount of time that it requires (which will vary beyond the confines of the seven-day week) to recover from the stress of exercise. The measurement/recovery method is out of date with the new model of fitness. Perhaps a more accurate measurement would be to start at "A" units of time, and then every time that an individual grows stronger, assume that it will simply take more units of time for full recovery—and then over-compensation or adaptation—to take place. Training within the confines of a week works well for beginners but not because it is a two-day or seven-day interval, but because the beginner's recovery happens to fall into this realm of time—the advanced trainee's does not. In 1971 Arthur Jones made the statement in his *Nautilus Bulletin #2* that

> When anything is in limited supply, then it is simply common-sense practice to make the best-possible utilization of the quantity that is available—and when you are not sure just how much is available, it is equally good practice to use as little as necessary; in the field of exercise, the implication is clear—use your limited recovery ability as wisely as possible, and as little as possible in line with the actual requirements for producing the results you are after.

This is absolutely true. And as your limited supply of recovery ability does not get bigger, but the demands you are placing on your muscles and energy systems do, it only stands to reason to disturb your limited reserve of recovery resources as sparingly as possible by training only as much as is required—not as many times as you can fit into an arbitrary time period such as seven days.

Q: One of the strength coaches at my university has the football players training with plyometrics, where they jump with weights and perform their repetitions as quickly as possible to become explosive. What are your thoughts on this method of training for golfers? Will it make me more explosive off the tee?

A: The facts of the matter regarding impact forces and the nature of muscle fiber recruitment obviously fly in the face of what some of the bodybuilding and strength coaches have been preaching regarding plyometrics and other such "explosive" movements for developing

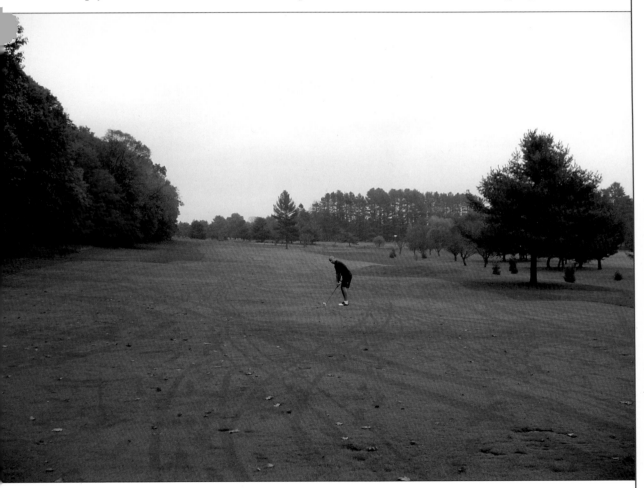

Make your body stronger through proper strength training—and then take that stronger you onto the course and play golf. Trying to train "explosively" will only lead to excess forces being placed on your joints and connective tissues, and could well result in your missing golfing opportunities because of needlessly incurred injuries.

strength and muscle size. Their theories, that the "fast-twitch" muscle fibers can only be activated by performing various exercises as fast as you possibly can, have been shown to be fallacious in light of what science has revealed regarding the principles of motor control and muscle fiber recruitment. First off, if you train utilizing a very high rate of speed and ballistic movements, you will be forced to use light weights as, the heavier the resistance, the slower you can move it. If you use a light weight, the brain immediately picks up on the FORCE required to move that weight and, obviously, with a light weight, the FORCE required to move the resistance at a high speed would prove sufficient to engage the "S" (slow twitch) and maybe the "FO" (fast oxidative or intermediate twitch) fibers. The "FG" (fast-twitch glycolytic) fibers—the ones most important to high speed movement and the one's contributing the most to increases in size and strength—are never activated in such a system because the resistance you will have restricted yourself to using will not be sufficient to warrant the brain sending the signal to recruit the "FGs" that would otherwise engage the full complement of muscle fibers. Not only does ballistic or plyometric training not stimulate the muscle fibers its theory purports it does, but it only involves half of the muscle fibers available to be stimulated in any given set. Obviously if you're only stimulating half the fibers you could be, your training system is only half as efficient as it could be, and certainly only half as efficient as Max Contraction Training, which engages all of the available muscle fibers (right down to the FG fibers). Any training system that is predicated on heaving weights up and down ballistically will not even come close to bringing the target muscle group into a position of full-muscular contraction for any meaningful length of time and certainly will not engage anywhere near the full complement of available muscle fibers. As if that wasn't enough, such training is highly traumatic to your joints and connective tissues. A barbell weighing 100 pounds, for example, if curled slowly in the conventional fashion will provide 100 pounds of resistance both concentrically and eccentrically (up and down). Holding 100 pounds in a position of full muscular contraction will do likewise. However, jerking and heaving that same 100-pound barbell up and down will magnify the trauma force on the joints to well over 1,000 pounds—and the impact to the joints which must suddenly stretch and then ballistically extend muscles, tendons, ligaments, and muscle fascia, can quickly add up to injury. Again, high-speed training is dangerous and far less productive than Max Contraction Training.

Q: I've heard that isometric type exercises can cause an increase in blood pressure. If so, doesn't this make Max Contraction and other "static" type exercise protocols more dangerous than regular training?

A: The truth is that your blood pressure goes up during any vigorous exercise of any sort, including cycling, cross-country skiing, running, calisthenics, and weight training. In the textbook entitled *Exercise Physiology* by Professors William D. McArdle, Frank I. Katch, and Victor L. Katch, they tested isometric or "motionless" exercise against two modes of isotonic exercise. The study was conducted at the University of Massachusetts and the blood pressure of normotensive subjects was measured directly with a pressure transducer connected to a catheter that was inserted into the femoral artery. They then tested the blood pressure response of the subject performing four sets of isometric bench

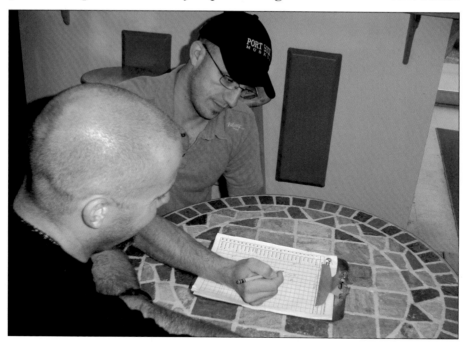

Max Contraction training is actually less risky than other forms of exercise.

presses at 25, 50, 75, and 100 percent of maximal voluntary contraction in the same arm and body position as the two other protocols, which were free weight bench presses performed at 25 and 50 percent of the maximum voluntary contraction and a hydraulic resistance bench press performed "all-out" for twenty seconds' duration at two settings: slow (for eleven reps) and fast (for sixteen reps) carried through a full range of motion.

According to the textbook, all three forms of exercise produced dramatic elevations in blood pressure—even with relatively light exercise that required only 25 percent of the maximal effort. In looking over the data myself, I note that the peak systolic and peak diastolic conditions were actually somewhat higher with the full range exercises than with the isometric exercise (at 100 percent contraction isometrically, the peak systolic was 225 and the peak diastolic was 156, compared with 232 and 154 for the free weight full-range bench press and 245 and 160 for the hydraulic full range bench press). This makes sense, of course, because it doesn't take a maximal effort to cause an increase in blood pressure. In fact, your blood pressure is probably rising right now from the sodium in the soft drink you're drinking. Many common everyday tasks like carrying a briefcase and maintaining your posture are largely static or isometric and not considered "dangerous."

It's interesting to note that the increase in blood pressure from full-range weight training was one of the reasons that Arthur Jones designed his Nautilus equipment the way he did and why he also stressed that you should not grip the handles of the machines too tightly when training. This is not to trivialize the concern—it is important that anyone beginning a vigorous weight training program get his or her physician's okay beforehand. But it's also a fact that any increase in blood pressure from weight training exercise such as Max Contraction returns to normal quite quickly after you complete your workout provided that your cardiovascular system is functioning normally. James Wright, Ph.D., in an article on motionless exercise—the same one that premiered my training system to North American audiences back in 1992—wrote that isometrics or "static" exercise did not cause blood pressure increases that were any greater than conventional forms of weight training, writing:

. . . there is no evidence that the transient elevations that occur during [isometric] exercise persist or influence the development of hypertension or cardiovascular risk. . . . the blood pressure changes are no more—and no different—than those that occur during any kind of heavy lifting. That's one reason some physicians in years past weren't too keen on weightlifting and bodybuilding. But who can say that transient elevations in blood pressure—which only require the heart, which is a muscle, to pump harder for a brief period—is bad for you?

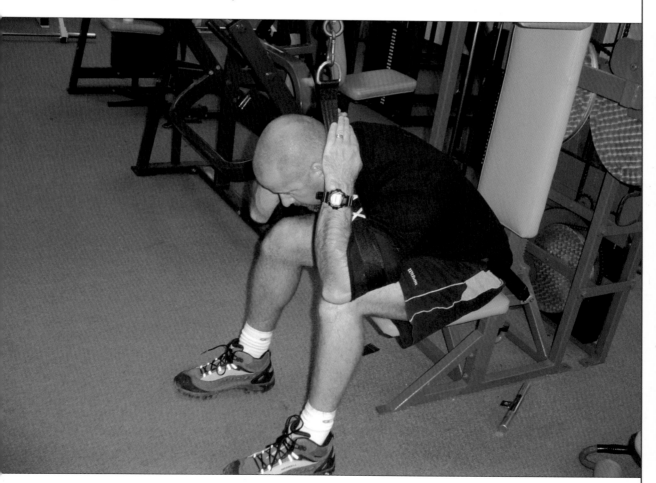

The idea that you can remove fat from one area of the body, such as the waist, by exercising it is a myth.

This said, individuals with a precondition to heart disease would obviously be at risk by engaging in any activity that elevates blood pressure—from swimming to weight training. And if you are one of these people, then Max Contraction Training would not be a wise thing to do—but it's no more dangerous and causes no greater increase in blood pressure than any other bodybuilding exercise. In fact, according to the study I just cited, it causes less of a blood pressure increase than conventional training.

Q: I would like to lose fat from the area around my chest and entire waist area without losing size anywhere else. Can I spot reduce these areas with Max Contraction?

A: Sorry to disillusion you, but "spot reduction" isn't physiologically possible; it is a bogus concept perpetrated by business interests selling "spot reduction" devices and supplements. When you go on a diet, fat will be mobilized from all of your body's multiple fat cells, not from isolated areas, such as those in the areas you might be exercising. Once fat has been broken down and mobilized it is transported by the blood to all the individual active cells in the body and burned for energy. You would be better advised to go on a general reducing diet in conjunction with Max Contraction Training, working all of your muscle groups in a single workout performed once to three times weekly. This will lower your overall percentage of body fat and build muscle at the same time, thereby causing a reduction in the areas you desire, while maintaining muscle size in all body parts.

Q: I like the idea of growing bigger and stronger muscles, but I've been told that should I ever stop training, all my muscles will turn to fat. What do you say to that?

A: I say that it's a supposition contrary to fact. Muscle and fat are two totally different types of tissue and one won't magically transform into the other any more than a peach will transform into a watermelon. Viewed under a microscope muscle is seen as long fibrous strands, known as myofibrils, while fat is comprised of little spherical globules. A chemical analysis of muscle and fat reveal the former to be made up of over 70 percent water, 6 percent lipids and about 22 percent protein. Fat, on the other hand is only 15 to 20 percent water, 70 percent lipids and approximately 15 percent protein. It's been a long standing false-hood that muscle turns to fat later in life, most likely arising from the

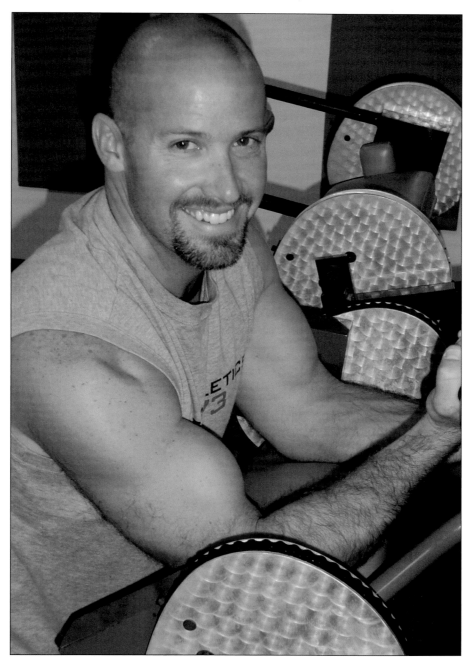

Muscle can't turn to fat anymore than a peach can turn into a watermelon; they are two different tissues.

fact that often times uneducated or just non-caring athletes would often continue eating the same quantity of food after they'd stopped competing as they did when they were competing. I knew many hockey players in Canada who were very lean when they were practicing several times a week and playing high-level hockey twice a week on top of this. Such a regimen required them to consume thousands of calories each day simply to maintain their bodyweight and fuel their training and game sessions. However, after their competitive careers ended they weren't nearly as active and thus didn't burn as many calories as they did when they were training and competing, with the result that a good many of them are now very fat. That doesn't mean that playing hockey will make you fat—and neither will bodybuilding training. As long as you match your calorie consumption to your energy expenditure, you needn't worry about your muscles "turning to" fat.

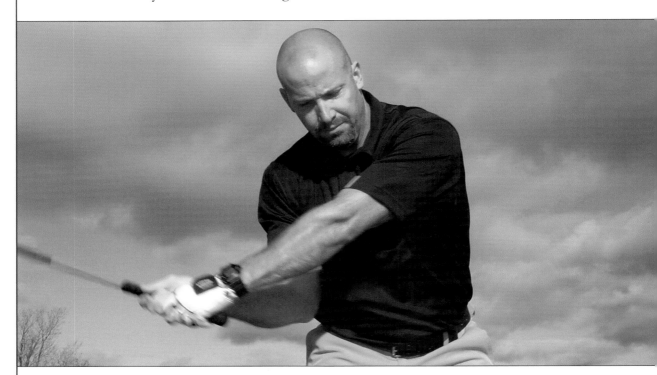

Train hard to stimulate a strength increase, allow enough time to recover and adapt, eat properly—and practice your skill set for the game of golf as often as possible. That's the most rational approach to improving your golf game.

SOURCES

BOOKS

Hatfield, Fred, *Bodybuilding: A Scientific Approach*. Chicago: Contemporary Books, 1988.

Lamb, David R. *Physiology of Exercise: Responses and Adaptations*. New York: MacMillan, 1984.

McArdle, William D., Frank I. Katch, and Victor L. Katch. *Exercise Physiology*. Philadelphia: Lea and Febiger, 1986.

Selye, Hans. *Stress Without Distress*. New York: New American Library, 1974.

Little, John, and Peter Sisco. *The Golfer's Two-Minute Workout*. New York: McGraw Hill, 1998.

JOURNALS

Berger, R. A. "Comparison of the effect of various weight training loads on strength." *Research Quarterly* 36:141–146, 1963.

Herbert, R. D., and M. Gabriel. "Effects of stretching before and after exercising on muscle soreness and risk of injury: systematic review." *British Medical Journal* 325:468–470, 2002.

Pope, R. P., R. D. Herbert, J. D. Kirwan, et al. "A randomized trial of preexercise stretching for prevention of lower-limb injury." *Medicine & Science in Sports & Exercise* 32:271–7, 2002.

Shrier, I. "Stretching before exercise does not reduce the risk of local muscle injury: a critical review of the clinical and basic science literature." *Clinical Journal of Sports Medicine* 9:221–227, 1999.

Thibault, M. C., et al. "Inheritance of human muscle enzyme adaptation to isokinetic strength training." *Human Heredity* 36 (6):341–7, 1986.

ONLINE REFERENCES

http://saveyourself.ca/articles/stretching.php
http://saveyourself.ca/bibliography.php?her00
http://news.bbc.co.uk/2/hi/health/2221716.stm
http://seriousstrength.com/flexibility.php
http://www.bmj.com/cgi/content/abstract/325/7362/468

ACKNOWLEDGMENTS

The author would like to thank both the Windermere Golf & Country Club and Muskoka Highlands (Muskoka, Ontario) for allowing us to photograph their beautiful courses. Also, the author would like to thank Jeremy Hymers for his participation in both the golf and exercise photo shoots. I would also like to acknowledge the hard work and contribution of two excellent trainers, particularly Cary Howe (who was extremely helpful during my two research projects at Nautilus North, and who is one of the best personal trainers on the planet) and Blair Wilson (who was the first to test the effects of hockey practice and competition on body composition and thus open a new window through which to view the training requirements of athletes during the competitive season). The understanding of the principles espoused in this book by the three individuals mentioned above have made the author's life much easier, as well as the lives of the thousands of clients they have trained throughout the years.

ABOUT THE AUTHOR

For over twenty years, John Little has worked alongside sports' greatest fitness authorities, athletes, champions, and innovators—from Steve "Hercules" Reeves, Jackie Chan, and Arnold Schwarzenegger, to six-time Mr. Olympia Dorian Yates and high-intensity training pioneer Mike Mentzer. In addition, Little and his wife, Terri, are the owners of Nautilus North Strength & Fitness Centre (www.nautilusnorth.com), which *Ironman* magazine lauded as "one of the leading fitness research centers in North America." Little is a regular columnist for *Ironman* and the innovator of three revolutionary training protocols (Max Contraction Training, Static Contraction Training, and Power Factor Training). His articles are published in every major fitness publication throughout the world, and he has written more than thirty books on bodybuilding, martial arts, history, and philosophy. Little's methods have been called "revolutionary" by the bodybuilding community.